CERVICAL CANC

CW01621485

CERVICAL CANCER
and how to stop worrying about it

Judith Harvey BM, BCh, DPhil
Sue Mack MA, CQSW
and
Julian Woolfson MB, ChB, MRCOG

faber and faber
LONDON · BOSTON

First published in 1988
by Faber and Faber Limited
3 Queen Square, London WC1N 3AU

Photoset by Parker Typesetting Service Leicester
Printed in Great Britain by
Richard Clay Ltd Bungay Suffolk
All rights reserved

© J. Harvey, S. Mack, J. Woolfson, 1988

British Library Cataloguing in Publication Data

Harvey, Judith
Cervical cancer – and how to stop worrying about it.
1. Cervix uteri —— Cancer
I. Title II. Mack, Sue II. Woolfson, Julian
616.99'466 RC280.U8

ISBN 0-571-14984-7

Contents

Acknowledgements

We have been helped and encouraged by our colleagues, friends and patients and are grateful to them all. We are particularly indebted to Jenny Aps, Gary Bradley, Dave Eastham and Monica Turner as well as those patients who have allowed us to use their comments.

Chapter 1
Introduction

Cancer of the cervix is a disease on the increase. Its toll has been 2000 British women a year. Now that number is set to rise sharply, and many of those at risk are young women. Women with small children. Women who have not yet had their children.

Cancer of the cervix is a preventable disease. The test which detects the disease at its pre-cancer stage is simple, cheap, painless and efficient. The treatment which removes the pre-cancer cells and so prevents cancer from developing is simple, painless and effective.

In theory, the test and the treatment are available to everyone. In practice, women are slipping through the net. Some do not know about the test, some are too embarrassed or frightened to be tested. Some want the test but find it difficult to get it. And some have the test and are not properly followed up. For some of these women the price they pay is their lives.

Like AIDS, cervical cancer has suddenly become a major health threat. Like AIDS, cervical cancer kills and like AIDS it is linked with sexual activity. Therefore, like AIDS it may arouse fear and guilt. Unless a cure is found, we shall have to change our sexual habits to prevent an epidemic of both diseases. But unlike AIDS, cervical cancer can be diagnosed and treated before it has done any damage. Even now, no one need die from it.

Now is a critical time for cervical cancer. Enough is known

that many women could be prevented from developing the disease, and those who do could all be cured. But only if everyone knows enough about it.

That is why we have written this book. In the following chapters we describe what cervical cancer is, how it develops, who is at risk, how it is diagnosed at a pre-cancerous stage and treated, and how it can be prevented. Because the idea of cancer is frightening we discuss the anxieties and problems that the disease presents, and suggest how they may be coped with. We hope that this information will help both individuals and society to ensure that women now and in the future do not have to suffer and die from cervical cancer.

Chapter 2
What is cervical cancer and pre-cancer?

It's easier to understand the meaning of smear tests and what is happening when you have treatment if you know a bit about the anatomy of the cervix and what is going on in the cells. In this chapter we explain where and what the cervix is and we look at how pre-cancer and cancer develop, as well as other common diseases of the cervix.

What is your cervix?

Your cervix (pronounced *sir-vix*) is part of your uterus (womb). As Figure 2/1 shows, the uterus is like a balloon. It has a part which can expand during pregnancy and a neck through which things can get in and out. The neck, which is the cervix, sits at the top of the vagina and so anchors the uterus to the rest of the body. It is firm and fleshy and about three centimetres (cm) across; the channel through it is called the endocervical canal. The canal is about the size of a pencil lead which is big enough to let the blood escape during a period. In the first stage of labour the contractions of the muscle of the rest of the uterus pull open the cervix until it is 'fully dilated' – wide enough to let the baby come through.

The cervix is the part of the uterus which can be examined directly. A doctor doing an internal examination can reach it with the tip of the fingers and it is possible to feel one's own cervix this way, although not always easy unless you are relaxed

Fig. 2/1 Anatomy of the uterus and cervix

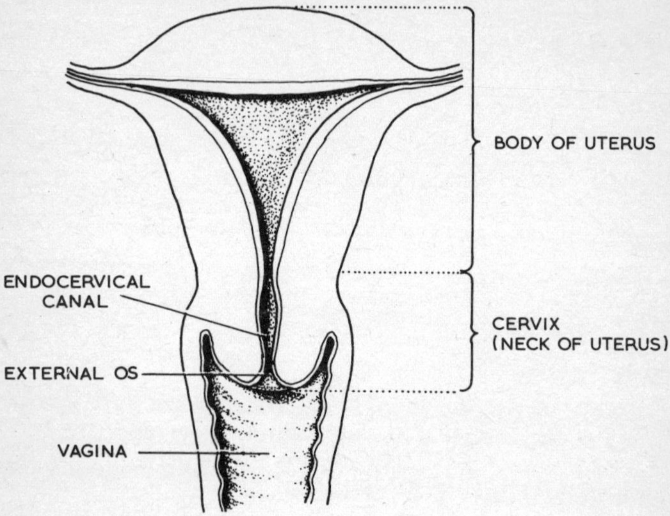

and have long fingers. If you insert your fingers into your vagina you will feel the flexible walls of the vagina around them. If you can reach far enough, at the top of the vagina you will encounter something that feels a bit like the end of your nose – firm but not hard and somewhat movable. That is the cervix. The canal is normally too small to feel but you may detect a slight dent in the middle like a button on a cushion. The opening is in the dent (Fig. 2/2).

The cervix resembles a cushion in that it is made of a thin outer covering filled with stuffing. The stuffing is mostly fibres with some muscle and blood vessels. The covering, or epithelium (pronounced *eppy-theel-ium*) is made of a sheet of cells. The part of the cervix which can be felt at the top of the vagina is covered with the same tough moist epithelium which lines the vagina. This is called squamous epithelium (pronounced *squaymus*). The endocervical canal through the cervix is lined with glands so its epithelium is called glandular epithelium. The junction between the two sorts of epithelium is called the 'transformation zone' because it is where the glandular epithelium is

Fig. 2/2 The cervix

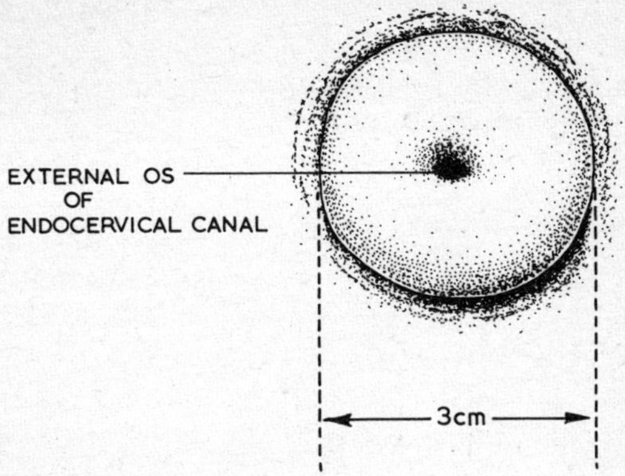

transformed into squamous epithelium. The transformation zone is very important and is usually just at the outside end of the endocervical canal (Fig. 2/3).

Fig. 2/3 The transformation zone

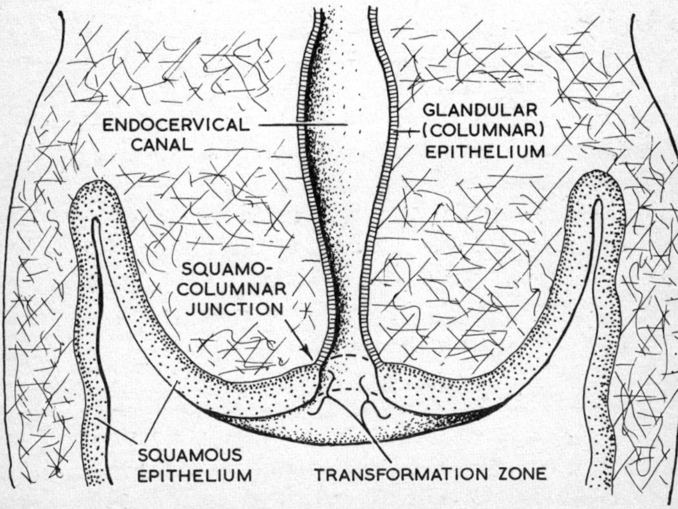

What does the cervix do?

Normally the cervix does nothing very obvious. The glandular epithelium produces sticky secretions which you notice only at times when they naturally increase – the middle of the month, or during pregnancy.

What about cancer?

The cells of the body are programmed to do different things according to where they are. So stomach cells produce digestive juices, muscle cells contract, nerve cells send signals. Like workers on any production line, the cells are kept under very strict control and not allowed to wander about. If cells escape from control they put their energy into multiplying. If that's all that goes wrong, a lump may form, but not too much harm is done. It is 'benign'. If, in addition, the production line is disrupted and the abnormal cells break out and spread around the body producing satellite factories and causing trouble, they have become 'malignant'. That is cancer.

What makes cells go out of control? Radiation, some chemicals, and viruses, and probably many other things, are 'carcinogenic' – help to cause cancer. But, like a seed starting to grow in soil, it seems that several different factors, which vary from cancer to cancer, are needed to trigger cells to behave abnormally.

What about cancer of the cervix?

Like any other organ the cervix can develop a cancer. The cells of the cervix which seem to be most vulnerable to carcinogens are those along the transformation zone. That may be because the cells here are changing from one type – glandular epithelium – to another – squamous epithelium.

The first changes towards cancer are microscopic – just a few abnormal cells in the epithelium. Given time, more and more cells may become abnormal. Given more time, some of these cells invade the bulk of the cervix and then the surrounding organs. This is the cancer that most people understand.

It is worth looking at this process in more detail because it explains why cervical cancer is a preventable disease.

The following illustrations (Figs. 2/4, 2/5 & 2/6) show what the epithelium of the cervix and the area immediately underneath it look like if you cut through it and put a thin slice under the microscope.

Fig. 2/4 A normal cervix

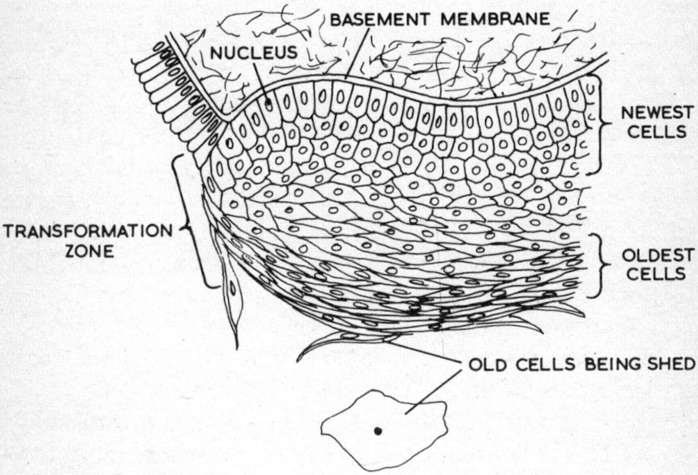

The squamous epithelium, which is about as thick as a piece of paper, is very like skin. It consists of cells packed in layers. In the middle of each cell is the nucleus containing the chromosomes which control its activity.

The bottom layer of cells sits on a sort of blanket called the basement membrane. This layer of cells divides and new cells are pushed up into the layers above. The cells get older and flatter as they rise towards the surface where they are rubbed off. The same process goes on in skin, and the cells that are shed form skin scales or dandruff.

Under the basement membrane the bulk of the cervix consists of fibres with some muscle cells and blood vessels.

The change which shows that cells are becoming cancerous is

Fig. 2/5 A cervix with pre-cancer

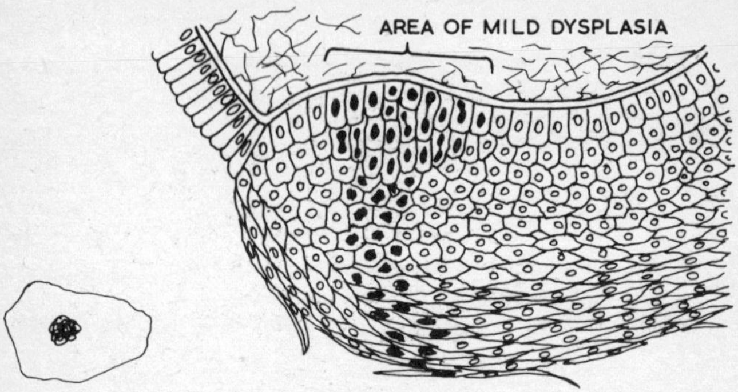

called dysplasia (pronounced *dis-plays-ya*). Instead of neat layers of similar cells, the cells become variable in size and shape, and they no longer form regular rows. Some cells can be seen dividing.

If these changes occur mostly in the bottom layers just above the basement membrane, the dysplasia is *mild*. If more of the layers are affected, it is *moderate*. If all the cells are abnormal, the dysplasia is *severe*.

Dysplasia isn't true cancer because the cells, though abnormal, are still in the right place. But it can go on to become true cancer, and every cervical cancer has gone through a period of dysplasia first. Dysplasia can therefore be called *pre-cancer*. It is also known, technically, as CIN or Cervical Intraepithelial Neoplasia (intraepithelial = within the epithelium or above the basement membrane; neoplasia = abnormal growth). CIN I, II and III correspond to *mild*, *moderate* and *severe* dysplasia.

If the dysplasia is severe enough, in time some of the abnormal cells will break through the basement membrane. They have then become malignant. At this stage there is *true* cancer.

If the cells have invaded only a little way, they don't do enough damage to be detectable except under the microscope and that stage is therefore called *micro-invasive* cancer.

With time, the abnormal cells will spread through the bulk of the cervix. Eventually and if the disease is not treated, the

Fig. 2/6 A cervix with true cancer

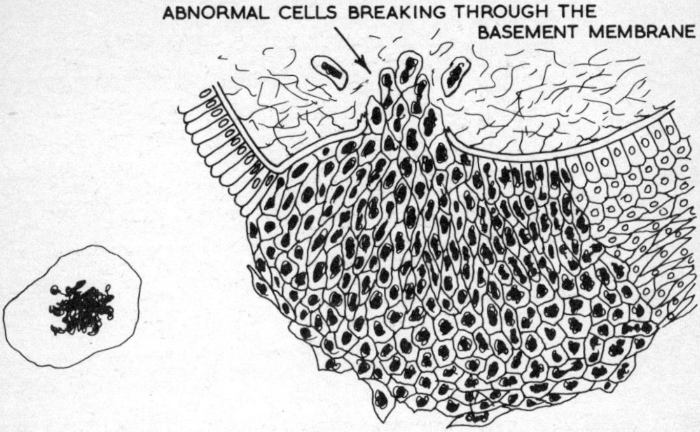

invasion will go further. Malignant cells from the cervix appear in the rest of the uterus and then around it. Eventually other nearby organs such as the bladder and bowels are affected. That is *advanced* cancer.

How long do these changes take?

Pre-cancer may progress from mild dysplasia to moderate and then to severe over the course of up to 20 years. Eventually the malignant cells may invade and produce a micro-invasive cancer, maybe more than 20 years after the start of the process. The true cancer then starts spreading, and that may take a few years to become advanced.

It is as if the disease progresses along a pathway from mild pre-cancer to more severe forms and then to true cancer. However, the progress is not inevitable. The disease can stop at any stage and never get any worse. It can even go backwards and clear up as if it had never been. The earlier the stage of the disease the more likely this is to happen. It is not known why the disease should stop in its tracks in this way.

Very rarely, the disease progresses very much faster than the normal 10 to 20 years, and again it is not clear why. This is discussed further in Chapter 3.

What is the significance of pre-cancer?

The significance is vital! The reason cancer is so hard to cure is that the malignant cells are so destructive and they become scattered around the body. In the pre-cancer stage, the cells are still contained and doing no harm. If that stage can be recognised, it is easy to treat and then cancer doesn't develop. The smear test, which tests for pre-cancer, and the treatment of pre-cancer, are described in the later chapters of the book.

Can you summarise all that?

See Fig. 2/7

Is there only one sort of cervical cancer?

There is only one common sort, that which develops in the transformation zone as described above, which to be absolutely correct is called 'squamous carcinoma of the cervix' (carcinoma = cancer). Very occasionally, cancer develops in the glandular tissue of the canal through the cervix. It is called 'adenocarcinoma of the cervix' and like the more common sort it has a pre-cancer phase and in most other ways behaves in a similar manner. It is only under the microscope that the difference can be seen.

The main significance of adenocarcinoma is that it probably is not caused by the things that cause the common cancer. They will be discussed in the next chapter.

Is cancer the only disease of the cervix?

No, definitely not. Common problems which the cervix can develop are what are often called *erosions*, and infections causing *cervicitis*.

What is a cervical erosion?

Occasionally the glandular lining spreads out of the canal and replaces some of the squamous epithelium on the vaginal sur-

Fig. 2/7 Flow chart summarising the changes of a cancer of the cervix

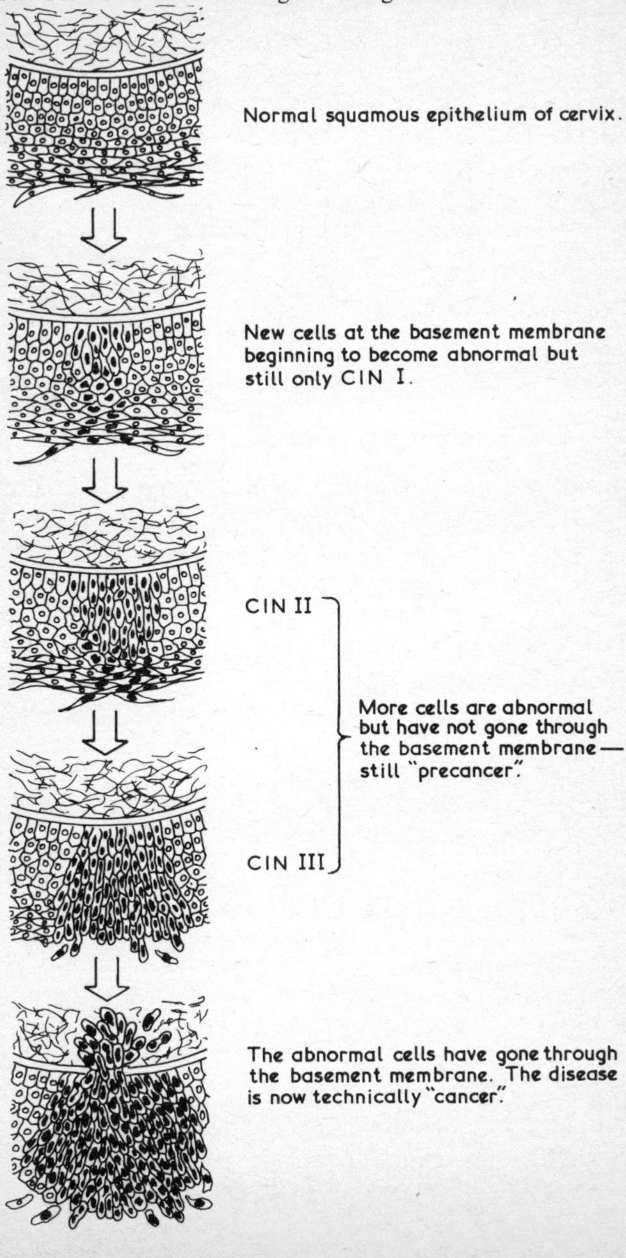

Fig. 2/8 Ectropion

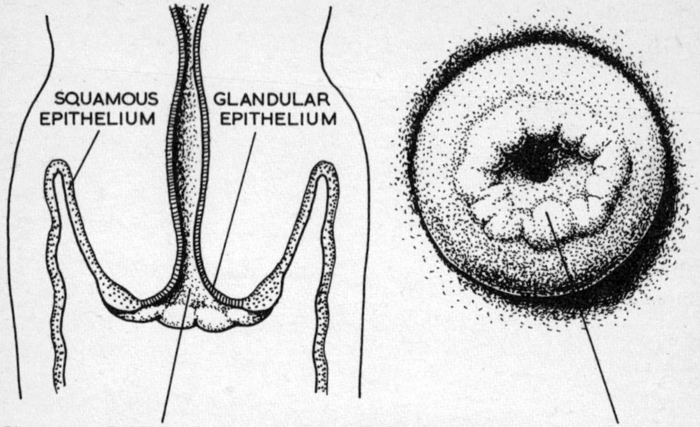

face of the cervix. This may happen when hormone levels are changing a lot – at puberty, during pregnancy, or while on the oral contraceptive pill: it is called *cervical ectropion*, or, more commonly but not strictly correctly, an *erosion*. Despite the name 'erosion', an ectropion isn't dangerous, but it can be a nuisance because the extra glandular tissue can produce excessive secretion. Furthermore, glandular tissue is not as tough as the usual covering and it more easily gets infected, causing more, and sometimes smelly, discharge. It may be damaged, especially by intercourse, causing bleeding. Ectropions (Fig. 2/8) tend to go away once puberty is over, or the baby is born, or if you stop taking the Pill.

More rarely a bare patch appears in the epithelium of the cervix as a result of damage due to long-standing infection. That is a genuine erosion and is best treated by cautery (freezing or burning).

What is cervicitis?

If your cervix becomes infected, you develop cervicitis (pronounced *service-itis*). You may not notice anything, but cervicitis can cause increased discharge which may smell unpleasant.

Vaginal infections can cause the same, and some vaginal and cervical infections are dangerous because they can spread up into the uterus and the tubes. Infection there can lead to sterility so it is important that possible infections are properly investigated and treated.

These minor diseases of the cervix are occasionally troublesome to the sufferer, but they do not lead to cancer.

In this chapter, we have described what cancer is and how it develops in the cervix. The next chapter looks at why it develops.

Chapter 3
Who is at risk?

If a weed is to grow, it needs strong seed and the right soil and weather. It won't grow in every garden all the year. Once it is established, it will eventually grow big enough to force out the flowers around it, and it will spread by seed all over the garden unless someone does some weeding in time. Cervical cancer behaves very like a weed. In this chapter the conditions needed for the 'seed' of cancer to 'germinate' are examined.

We do not know enough to be able to predict for certain whether someone will or won't develop cancer. But if we look at the women who do develop pre-cancer or cancer and compare them with women who don't, we can see that there are differences between the two groups. It seems that these differences, in what women are, or do, or take, in some way make them more likely to develop cervical cancer.

These differences, or risk factors, relate to infection with wart virus, to sexual activity, to smoking and to taking the Pill, and possibly to pregnancy.

What is the significance of warts?

It has been known for some while that a variety of cancers are caused by cells becoming infected with viruses and it is probable that cervical cancer is one of them.

The virus incriminated in cervical cancer is the *wart* virus. It is also known as Human Papilloma Virus or HPV for short, and it has many different forms. Those which affect the cervix are different from those which cause the familiar warts on the hands and elsewhere.

As described in Chapter 2, the part of the cervix where the glandular tissue which lines the endocervical canal changes to the squamous epithelium which lines the vagina is called the transformation zone. The cells of the transformation zone are particularly vulnerable to attack from the cervical wart virus. It gets into the cells and causes changes in them. The signs of these changes can be seen when infected cells are examined under the microscope.

HPV doesn't automatically lead to cancer, but it seems that cells which have been affected by it are vulnerable, in a way that uninfected cells are not, to other influences which, in combination, trigger the cancerous change. HPV is necessary, but not sufficient, for the development of cancer.

How does one catch warts?

From someone else. Cervical HPV also affects the penis. Infected men may or may not develop visible warts, but even if they are invisible they can pass the virus to their sexual partners. And that leads on to the next risk factor, sexual activity.

What is the link between sex and cervical cancer?

It is almost certain that cervical cancer is a sexually transmitted disease.

It has been known for a long time that cervical cancer is much commoner in women who have many sexual partners, and less common in nuns, lesbians and societies where there is very little sex outside marriage. It seems logical that a woman with many sexual partners is more likely by chance to encounter someone with HPV.

However, a lot of women who have only ever had one partner develop cervical cancer. But the key is that their partners have at some time had another sexual relationship.

So it is men's promiscuity just as much as women's which puts women at risk. But why? The more partners anyone, male or female, has had, the more likely they are to have picked up HPV and so to be endangering themselves or their partners. A woman may be faithful all her life to one partner but if he has at any time, perhaps long before he met her, had one sexual encounter with someone with HPV, she is at risk.

Does circumcision make any difference?

Warts often grow under the foreskin, so it's easier to know whether or not a man has warts if he's circumcised. Apart from that, probably no.

What makes the cervix more easy for the virus to attack?

Two things seem to: hormones and smoking.

What about hormones?

We know that when levels of female hormones are undergoing great changes at times such as puberty and pregnancy, the transformation zone is particularly vulnerable to HPV.

The same conditions can lead to cervical ectropion ('erosion'), but an ectropion itself isn't dangerous and doesn't lead to cancer.

The statistics show that women who start having sex at a young age are more likely to develop cervical cancer than those who don't have intercourse until their late teens or early twenties. Not only is their cervix more easily attacked, but they may well have more partners and be more likely to pick up HPV.

Another aspect of cervical cancer in very young women is that it seems to progress faster from mild to severe dysplasia and then to full cancer. This is probably also a consequence of the dramatic changes of puberty, and a very worrying one.

What about the Pill?

Women who take the Pill for five or ten years are probably

slightly more likely to develop dysplasia. Other things are much more important and as long as you are happy with the Pill and have regular checks you are most unlikely to come to any harm. But if you are worried, discuss it with your doctor.

What about smoking?

Women who smoke are eight times more likely to develop cervical cancer than equivalent non-smokers. That's a big increase in risk.

The cancer-causing chemicals in cigarette smoke do their damage to the lungs but they don't stop there. They are absorbed into the bloodstream and are spread all over the body, damaging most of the tissues they pass through. Cancer of the lung and of the cervix are not the only cancers that are more common in smokers.

Are any other things linked with cervical cancer?

First, social and economic status. The figures show that less advantaged women are two or three times more likely to develop the disease than those who are better-off. That is after allowing for differences in sexual and smoking habits.

Exactly why this should be isn't clear, but the same is true of almost every disease except, oddly, breast cancer which is more common in professional women. Generally poorer health may play a role.

A second possible link is with seminal fluid. There may be some factor in semen which encourages cervical cells to become pre-cancerous. It may be the chromosomes of the sperm themselves; no one is sure yet.

The connection between cervical cancer and the wart virus has only been known for a few years. Research is going on, in the laboratory and in the community, and in the future it is likely that links will be discovered with more factors in our bodies, our habits and our environment.

Are other vaginal infections linked with cervical cancer?

Some vaginal infections are spread by sexual contact, just as HPV is, so someone who has HPV may have another infection as well. But that doesn't mean that other infections help to cause cancer.

It used to be thought that the virus which causes genital herpes also caused cervical cancer. We are now less certain exactly what the link is. It may be just coincidence.

There is nothing to suggest that *thrush* (Candida) makes you more likely to develop cervical cancer.

What about diet and race and occupation?

These are certainly important risk factors in some cancers. A low fibre diet makes bowel cancer more likely. Stomach cancer is more common in Japanese. Men who work with dyestuffs are at risk of cancer of the bladder. But as long as you are generally healthy, and that involves eating a good diet, there is no convincing evidence that any of these factors makes a difference in cancer of the cervix.

Can cervical cancer be set off by an emotional crisis?

Many cancer sufferers relate the start of their disease to a crisis in their life – the death of a loved one, a car crash, losing their job. It is difficult to prove. It is equally difficult to disprove.

Maybe in time we shall understand much more about the part emotions play in causing cancer. Till then, all we can say is that it is possible, but other factors come first.

Can you summarise the risk factors?

Yes, but remember that all the risk factors say is that people with them are *more* likely to develop cancer than those without. It's impossible to say for certain that any woman will, or won't, develop cervical cancer. It certainly is not just disadvantaged women who smoke, take the Pill and have lots of partners.

Many women who don't fit that picture at all are found on smear testing to have developed dysplasia. But if you were to stop women in the street, you would find that more of those with risk factors than those without had dysplasia. As in betting, the 100:1 outsider wins the race now and again, but the one with the shortest odds is the favourite.

What about adenocarcinoma of the cervix?

We do not yet know what causes this sort of cervical cancer. It does not appear to be passed on by sexual contact or as yet to be linked to any of the other risk factors associated with the commoner disease. But it sometimes occurs and it is getting more common. That is one reason why every woman is potentially at risk and should have regular smear tests.

Smear tests are described in the next two chapters.

Chapter 4
How is pre-cancer discovered?

In the previous chapter we described how cells of the cervix can become dysplastic, or pre-cancerous, and how there is a spectrum of increasing severity of dysplasia which turns into true cancer when the abnormal cells break through the basement membrane and invade the surrounding tissue.

Dysplasia itself does no harm. The problem is that if it is left it stands a high chance of becoming invasive.

Dysplasia can be cured by destroying the abnormal cells. If it is cured, the danger of cancer disappears.

The saddest thing is that dysplasia causes no symptoms. There is nothing to make a woman suspect that she has dysplasia. That is why the smear test is so important.

What is the smear test?

The smear test is a simple way of identifying dysplasia. It allows the screening of a large number of women to find who has pre-cancer, so it can be treated before it develops into true cancer. It was devised by Dr George Papanicolaou and is called the Pap test in the USA.

As described in Chapter 2, the cervix is constantly making new cells from the bottom layer of its covering and losing them from the top. If there is dysplasia, some of the cells which are shed will be abnormal. If some of those cells can be collected and examined under the microscope, it is possible to diagnose dysplasia even though it causes no symptoms.

The test involves rubbing some of the cells off the surface of the cervix with a flat wooden stick called a spatula. The cells are then transferred to a glass microscope slide by wiping the spatula on the slide. The slide is labelled, put in preserving fluid and sent to the local pathology laboratory where it is processed and stained to show up the cells. The cytologist (pronounced *site-ologist*), a specially trained technician who is often a doctor, examines each slide under a microscope.

Fig. 4/1 The smear test

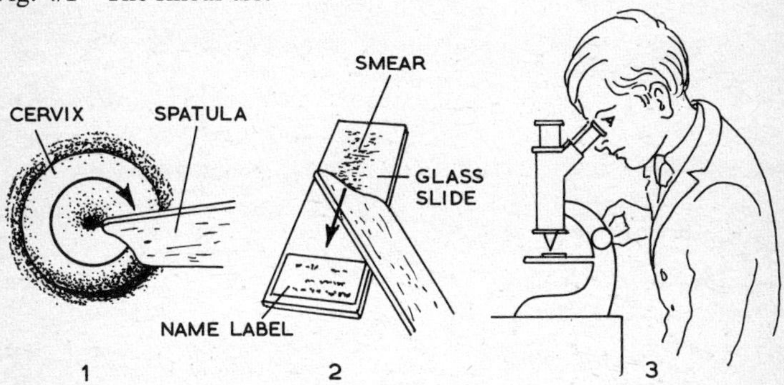

What does the smear test show?

The cytologist sees a scatter of cells. Some will be normal, some may have wart virus changes and some may have abnormalities characteristic of dysplasia. Like an archaeologist working out what a wall was like from a heap of fallen stones, the cytologist can estimate how severe the dysplasia is, although it is never possible to tell whether cells from a slide suggesting severe dysplasia are actually invading the basement membrane.

The smear test shows up both squamous cell carcinoma and adenocarcinoma in their pre-cancer stage. Women with pre-cancer can then be treated to avoid development of full cancer.

Is the smear test 100% reliable?

Unfortunately not – very few things ever are. But it is pretty good and if, as is now being recommended, the first smear test a woman has is repeated after a year, the number of pre-cancers missed would be very, very small.

Who should have smear tests?

Anyone who is at risk – and effectively that means all women. And they should be tested regularly. But to screen every woman every year would be very demanding of time and finance, as well as being unnecessary. Ideally every woman should be screened just often enough to catch new pre-cancers, but not more.

What are the current recommendations for screening?

The Department of Health and Social Security (DHSS) produced its guidelines in 1984. They are based on the traditional picture of cervical cancer as a very slow-growing disease of older women. They recommend that women have a smear once every five years from age 35 to 65, plus once during each pregnancy and otherwise only once or twice during their sexually active life.

That is better than nothing. But it is clear that this is now too little and too late to stop many women from developing a preventable cancer.

The age-group with the most dysplasia is the 25- to 35-year-olds so screening *must* cover women in this age-group effectively. And every five years is not often enough to catch every case before it becomes invasive.

How often is often enough?

The more often you screen, the fewer cases are missed. In the USA annual testing is recommended. But the difference between every year and every three years is a lot of work for very few more cancers prevented.

A big study of screening programmes in eight countries showed that the number of women developing cancer would be reduced to a very low level if all women had their first smear test soon after their first sexual intercourse, then a second test one year later, and then every three years until old age.

Many doctors in Britain try to follow that regime. But others stick to the old DHSS regulations, partly because they are only paid to do smear tests on women over 35. And the arrangements for doing tests and processing the results in this country is haphazard, to say the least.

The British Medical Association (BMA) produced a Report in 1986 and on the basis of all the research they recommended three-yearly testing from the age of 20. It is likely that pressure from doctors' and women's groups will persuade the Government to alter its policy. We sincerely hope so.

Would new recommendations eliminate cervical cancer?

They could. But only if they were put into practice.

It's one thing to recommend that every woman has a smear test every three years from the age of 20. It's another to make it happen.

There are three main problems. First, persuading all women to have the test; second, processing the slides; and third, ensuring that the results of the tests are acted upon.

The second problem, that of improved laboratory facilities, is a matter of money and organisation. Cervical screening is so important that we can expect resources to be made available. We hope it is in time.

The first problem is much more difficult. Do you know when your next smear is due? How many 20-year-olds are aware they should have a smear, and how many know where to go for one? And what about the women who 'won't' have a smear? We know from the figures that they are at most risk of cancer. How do we get them to the clinic?

The BMA Report of 1986 recommends that every health district should set up a system, rather like that for children's inoculations, for letting every woman know that she is due for a smear, for recording the result and informing the woman, and for checking that women with abnormal smears have received the appropriate further investigation. Computers are essential for this complicated task – so many different clinics do smear tests, so many people change their addresses. But it is quite possible, as one or two districts who have already computerised have proved.

Screening women who are reluctant to have the test is not easy. It is not enough to tell them when and where they should have the test. If they are too frightened, they won't go. They will not be persuaded by poster campaigns or newspaper advertisements. Few people would be in favour of making it illegal not to have a smear test. They need a more personal approach. The BMA Report suggests that health visitors and GPs are the people who can best reach women who otherwise wouldn't be tested. And we hope that information like this book may help to persuade some women that the benefits of having a smear test outweigh their fears.

As for the third problem, if all women received their result and the laboratories were able to check that abnormal smears had been followed up, we should have no more women dying of cancer after an abnormal smear.

To sum up, we need more than just suitable recommendations to crack the problem. Making screening effective requires a great deal of organisation and the money to do it and provide the laboratories and clinics to deal with the work. The Government is theoretically willing, but it needs pressure to make it happen: from the doctors; from the cancer prevention societies; from women's groups; from you and me.

Does the smear test reveal true cancer?

The purpose of the smear test is to detect the disease at its asymptomatic pre-cancer stage. A smear test may show that a woman already has true cancer but, ironically, a person with an invasive tumour may have a normal smear.

However, a cancer at that stage is probably making its presence felt in other ways. It is likely to cause bleeding, particularly after intercourse, and since a tumour easily becomes infected there may be a smelly discharge. There is rarely much pain until the disease is far advanced. These symptoms could be, and usually are, due to things which aren't cancer and which are easily put right.

If everyone had regular smear tests, no one would develop true cancer. Until then, it is important that women with worrying symptoms should go to the doctor. Gynaecologists would far rather see a clinic full of women with abnormal bleeding or discharge which turns out to be due to something very minor, than have people stay away and so miss the one woman with a cancer. The sooner it is diagnosed the more likely it is to be cured.

Chapter 5
Having a smear test

The purpose of a smear test – to detect dysplasia before it becomes true cancer – and what it is, have been described in Chapter 4. But knowing about the test and having it are rather different things. This chapter is all about having a smear test.

What does a smear test involve for me?

> *'I hate having internal examinations so it was a real effort to make myself go for the test, but I must admit that the smear itself was virtually painless.'*
>
> *'The doctor did my smear test during my postnatal check-up. I barely noticed it.'*

It would all be a lot simpler if the cervix were easier to get at! Since it is about 7.5cm inside at the top of the vagina, getting a good look at it, which is essential if an adequate smear test is to be done, involves an internal examination.

You will be asked to lie down, generally on your back with your legs drawn up and your knees apart. The doctor will then open up the vagina to see the cervix by inserting an instrument called a *speculum*. Although it is a bit uncomfortable it is not as bad as you might think if you have caught sight of the speculum beforehand – it has two rounded arms (which are moved apart once the speculum is inserted) attached to a ring through which the cervix can then be seen and it has to be said that it looks very medieval, particularly if it is made of metal!

The doctor will then, with the aid of a light, look through the speculum at your cervix and take the smear. It takes a few seconds and it is a bit like rubbing your nose with a lolly stick – you hardly feel it. And that is it.

Where can I get a smear test done?

> *'My friend had just had an abnormal smear and that frightened me. My GP wouldn't do a smear because I'm only 29. I got more and more worried until I found somewhere else to have it done.'*

Most GPs do smear tests. A Family Planning Clinic will test any woman who is registered at the clinic, and Well Woman Clinics, who are pleased to see anyone, do smear tests as a routine part of their service. Should you be attending an antenatal clinic or gynaecology out-patients, the staff will probably ask when you last had a smear test and if you are due for one it will be done.

It can be difficult to get a smear test, especially if your only option is the GP. *Don't* be put off by the GP's receptionist; ask to see the doctor to discuss it. If you are still getting nowhere, you will have to find somewhere else.

Any woman who has difficulty getting a smear test should telephone the Family Planning Association. They have 11 regional offices and a headquarters in London (where they are known as the Family Planning Information Service); the numbers are on page 83, as well as in the telephone directory. They will tell you the nearest place to get a smear test.

If it takes you a while to get your smear test, don't worry. Should you prove to have an abnormal smear, a delay of a few weeks or even months will not be dangerous: waiting for years is fatal.

I find the idea of a smear test very embarrassing!

You aren't alone! Almost all women, even if they have had numerous internal examinations, face another one with reluctance. It is somewhat undignified, somewhat uncomfortable and certainly very personal. But it is also life-saving.

If it helps, take a friend with you, or find a woman doctor (see below). When you are having the smear taken, try to relax yourself as much as possible because the more you can do so, the easier, quicker and less uncomfortable the procedure. Try to concentrate on your breathing – women who have had babies will know the trick. And remember that the doctor or nurse who is taking the smear does up to a dozen a day – and if they encountered someone who enjoyed having it done they would be most alarmed!

I should much prefer a woman doctor. Is that possible?

> *'The Practice nurse does all the smear tests at my GP's surgery. You don't have to see the doctor, and she was very gentle and reassuring.'*

Family Planning Clinics and Well Woman Clinics generally have women doctors; if you have a male GP but he has a woman partner, ask if you could see her for your smear. Alternatively, you may find that the nurse at your clinic or practice is trained to take smears. Do ask; you won't be the first person to have requested to see another woman for a smear.

Can a smear test be done when I have a period?

It's much better to put off a smear test until your period is finished because the bleeding, unless it is very light, makes the test difficult to do and the result difficult to interpret.

What if I am pregnant?

There is no problem about having a smear test when you are pregnant, but it isn't advisable to give treatment to pregnant women, so if your smear was abnormal you would have to wait for the next step. The few months' delay isn't a danger to your health or that of your baby, but of course it isn't pleasant to have it hanging over you. That's why some clinics suggest that if you are hoping to become pregnant in the near future, you should have a smear and get any treatment out of the way first.

I am disabled – is that a problem?

It may occasionally be a problem, but it is a soluble one! You and the doctor will be able to work out some position that makes it possible to take a smear in comfort.

If you can't get to the clinic or surgery your GP can probably take a smear at home, so ask.

Some of my friends refuse to have a smear

'What's the point of finding out – they can't do anything to cure cancer.'

Some people are very afraid of cancer and they may transfer their fears to the smear test. If they clearly understood that the test is not to show that they have cancer, but to detect abnormal cells which may lead to cancer so it can be prevented easily, they might overcome their fears.

Who should have smear tests?

In a word, everyone! As explained in the previous chapter, some women are more at risk than others, but cervical cancer can develop in absolutely any woman, so every woman should have a smear test every three years from her teens until old age.

When will the result of my smear test be available?

'I was horrified when they said it would take two months to get the result. Don't they realise how worrying it is?'

The laboratories have so many smear tests to examine that it may take several weeks or even a few months for the results to come through. This can be a worrying time, and there is a growing need for more facilities for analysing smear tests so that the results can be available much more quickly. But even if it takes 12 weeks, the delay isn't long enough to affect the progress of dysplasia, if you are one of the minority who has an abnormal smear.

How will I hear the result?

> *'I think they should let everyone know their result, whatever it is. Unless you actually know you're clear, you always have this thought at the back of your mind that it was abnormal but the result got lost in the post or something.'*

The laboratory sends the result to the doctor who took the smear. Different places make different arrangements for passing the result on to you, so ask the person who takes the smear when and how you will be informed.

Often, they will inform you of the result only if there is a problem. This arrangement saves on administration, but many women will worry until they hear for themselves that they have the all clear. In 1985 slip-ups occurred in the notification system in Oxford and several women with positive smears were not informed. Consequently they were not treated and they developed a full-blown cancer.

We therefore believe that everyone should be informed whatever the result. Unless your surgery undertakes to tell everyone, there are two things we recommend you to do:

First, ask for your result. Telephone or call in at your doctor's shortly after the result is due back from the laboratory.

Second, ask your surgery or clinic why they don't inform everyone and encourage them to do so. You could suggest a system similar to that operated by a general practice we know. The doctors undertake to contact everyone with an abnormal smear, but when a normal result comes back it is entered against the person's name on a list. The list is held by one member of the surgery team and all women know when, and how, in person or by phone, to contact her for the result. When a woman has her result, the list is ticked so the doctors can check who knows and who doesn't.

I'm very nervous about getting my result

> *'Five years ago I had an abnormal smear and needed treatment. I've had smear tests every year since then and I know they will almost certainly be OK, but I've been so frightened I've asked someone else to get the result for me. This year for the first time I felt able to ring them up myself.'*

Many people, particularly if they have had abnormal smears in the past, are afraid of bad news. Quite rightly, few surgeries would pass a result on to anyone else, but there is nothing to stop you taking someone else with you. Or, if they will post the result, it may be easier to read it or get someone else to open the letter for you. And remember, even if you do have an abnormal smear, it doesn't mean you have cancer. It means you can be treated to stop your developing it.

I don't understand the result and that worries me

The report on your smear test has two parts: first, a description of what the cells from your cervix looked like, and second, on the basis of the first part, a recommendation to the doctor about what should happen next. In the next chapter we describe all the possible results you might get.

The vast majority of smear tests are normal and nothing more needs to be done until your next test is due in three years' time.

A very few show obvious dysplasia and the report will recommend a clinic appointment for further investigation and treatment. If that happens to you, read Chapters 7 and 8 which describe what happens after you have an abnormal smear.

The problem arises when the results aren't clear-cut. If you aren't sure what's going on, this is what we suggest you do. Take a look at the next chapter so you have an idea of what the reports are all about, then make an appointment to see the doctor and take this book with you when you go. Ask to see the report and compare the report with the reports in Chapter 6. Then discuss it with your doctor. Usually, that will sort things out, but if you are still unhappy, you may have to ask the doctor to refer you to the specialist so that your mind can be put at rest.

I've had smear after smear and they keep saying 'repeat smear'

> *'You know if they tell you to have another smear in three months' time it's not right. I thought I had cancer and they didn't want to tell me.'*

This sometimes happens, for instance if some inflammation makes the smear difficult to interpret. In theory, it is simpler to repeat a smear than to refer you to the specialist, but it adds up to a lot of work in the long run, and more importantly, you have a cloud hanging over you for months and sometimes years.

If one smear shows inflammation, it is sensible to repeat it, but if the second or certainly the third is still the same, we feel you should have specialist examination and treatment to put an end to the worry.

For most women, the smear test is a bit of an ordeal, and the current arrangements in this country for doing the test don't make it any easier. The important thing to remember is that the aim of the test is not to show that you have cancer, but to see if you have a condition which may develop into cancer if it is left. And it is not going to be left. So a few minutes' embarrassment can save your life.

Chapter 6
The results of smear tests

The report on a smear test has two parts. First, it says what the cytologist saw under the microscope. Second, it recommends what should be done about it.

The first part is a straightforward description. The second part is tricky, because there is so much we have to learn about the way abnormalities of the cervix behave. The problem is to strike the right balance between referring anyone with any abnormality for treatment, in which case a lot of women would undergo unnecessary distress and the clinics would be unable to cope with the demand, and referring too few people, in which case some women would go on to develop a cancer which should have been prevented.

After much discussion, cytologists have drawn up a table of recommended reports. Most reports nowadays will follow the recommendations and the aim of this chapter is to list and explain all the possible reports.

Three-quarters of all smears are normal. Very few – 3% or less – show obvious dysplasia. The remainder do not give a satisfactory answer for a variety of reasons and generally need to be repeated.

Negative **Routine recall**

This means that nothing abnormal of any sort has been found, and you do not need any more attention until your next smear is due. As explained in Chapter 4, ideally that should be in three years' time. Some clinics will send you a reminder when you are next due for a smear but unfortunately it is often up to you to ask, so try to remember when you last had a smear and when your next one is due.

Inadequate or unsuitable **Repeat smear soon**

Not every smear is perfectly done – it isn't that easy. If there aren't sufficient cells for the pathologist to comment on, you should be asked to go for a repeat smear. A nuisance for you, but not a worry.

No endocervical cells seen **Repeat smear soon** (*or*) **Routine recall**

Endocervical cells are cells from the glandular lining of the cervical canal. If the cytologist sees endocervical cells he or she can be certain that there are also cells from the transformation zone of the cervix, which is important because it is there that dysplasia starts.

The cytologist may feel that the smear should be repeated to be sure that cells from the key area have been taken. But if there are plenty of cervical cells on the slide and they are all normal, he or she may be sufficiently happy that all is well to give you the all clear.

Inflamed **Repeat in 6 (or 12) months** (*or*) **Treat and repeat**

An infection can inflame your cervix and a smear may only remove debris from the infection. The smear needs to be repeated when the infection has subsided and a good smear can be done, but there is no urgency. The worse the infection, the longer it will take to clear. Some infections clear up on their own; severe ones may need antibiotics, which your doctor will prescribe.

The problem is that inflammation can linger and some women find themselves having smear after smear, which can be a great worry. As explained in the previous chapter, we think that after a second inflamed smear, a woman should be referred to a specialist. It is unlikely that she has cancer, but whatever is causing the inflammation is not going to clear up without expert attention.

Koilocytosis (*or*)	**Repeat in 3 (or 6) months then**
Warty changes (*or*)	**refer if still abnormal** (*or*)
Superficial dyskariosis	**Refer for colposcopy**

Koilocytes (pronounced *coil-o-sites*) are cells which show signs of wart virus infection. As explained in Chapter 3, wart virus infection is involved in the development of cancer. Not everyone who gets the infection develops cancer, and if cancer is going to develop it takes some years. That is why some laboratories suggest the smear is repeated, and if the signs of the infection go away, fine. But many cytologists recommend that a woman with wart virus infection should see a specialist at a colposcopy clinic after the first smear. It is more satisfactory to have expert investigation and treatment if it is needed than to have one not-quite-right smear after another.

Borderline (*or*)	**Repeat in 3 (or 6) months then**
Severe inflammation (*or*)	**refer if still abnormal** (*or*)
Mild dyskariosis	**Refer for colposcopy**

'Borderline' means the cells look slightly odd, but do not appear to be pre-cancerous. Cells with what the cytologists call dyskariosis (pronounced *dis-carry-osis*) have almost certainly come from a dysplasia. Mild, moderate and severe dyskariosis are more or less equivalent to mild, moderate and severe dysplasia. So mild dyskariosis suggests a very early pre-cancer. At this stage the abnormalities often go away with time – a repeat smear might be perfectly normal. But, as with the wart infection in the section above, it isn't possible at the moment to tell which case will go away and which will get worse, so many cytologists recommend you see a specialist earlier rather than later.

Moderate dyskariosis	**Refer for colposcopy**

This probably means there is a pre-cancer and most cytologists would refer you straight to the colposcopy clinic to find out for sure. Since this can also clear up of its own accord, in some places they will recommend another smear and not refer you unless that is abnormal, too.

Severe dyskariosis **Refer for colposcopy**

This is almost certainly pre-cancer and you need further tests, so you will be referred to the colposcopy clinic.

Dyskariotic endocervical cells/glandular **Refer for colposcopy**

If this, or something similar, appears on a report, it suggests that something is unusual about cells on the smear from the glandular canal through the cervix. You will be referred to the colposcopy clinic so that you can be investigated to check that you are not in the process of developing adenocarcinoma, the rarer form of cervical cancer.

We hope that we have covered all the possibilities, but if your report doesn't seem to fit into any of the categories listed above, and it isn't clear what is going on, ask your doctor to telephone the cytologist, preferably while you are there, to clarify the report. It is better to do that than to spend months worrying about it.

As you will have gathered, if you have read all the sample reports, it is easy if the smear test shows a clear 'no' – normal – or a clear 'yes' – looks like severe dysplasia. Everybody agrees on what to do about it. It is when the test shows the very early changes of dysplasia that the differences in policy are found.

The disease can at any stage get better of its own accord, and the earlier it is, the more often that happens. Unfortunately, the only way we know to tell which will get better and which will get worse is to wait and see. In the old days, further investigation meant an operation for everyone, so understandably doctors preferred to wait before doing anything. Now that we have colposcopy, further investigation and treatment are much easier and it is sensible to do it at a much earlier stage. What colposcopy is and what happens at a colposcopy clinic are described in Chapter 8.

Chapter 7
Having an abnormal smear test

For most women, the news that they have an abnormal smear is a shock. This chapter is to prepare women with an abnormal smear for the emotional problems it can bring.

Hearing the news

> *'The doctor rang me and said, "Your smear was not quite normal", and I never heard another word she said.'*
>
> *'I just wanted him to get off the phone so that I could ring Mum.'*
>
> *'He kept talking about treatment, but never mentioned cure.'*

Whether they receive the news by telephone, letter or in person, for many women the immediate shock of the words 'abnormal smear' is so frightening that they may be unable to hear anything else that is said.

You may immediately assume you have cancer. That will probably block out everything else. It is hard to listen to someone when you think you might be dying. Many women report that they could not understand, or were not given any information. This may sometimes be true, but it is also the case that some women just cannot listen to any more until they have had time to absorb the shock.

If you are told that you have an abnormal smear it may be helpful to make an appointment to see the doctor, nurse or counsellor in a few days. That will give you time to recover from the shock, think of all your questions and perhaps find someone to go with you. Taking a friend or relative not only gives you moral support but usually means that one of you will remember all the questions and, more importantly, the answers. If you have to go alone, or prefer to, write your questions down. It will help you and the person you are seeing to sort out what you want to know.

The doctor or nurse probably won't be able to give you detailed information at this stage. You will be having further tests and you will have to wait for the results of those. However, they should be able to explain in general terms what is happening to you and to help you cope.

Handling the stress

> *'Before she stopped talking I was working out who was going to look after my kids.'*

> *'I felt angry that there was something there. I was fit and well, but there was still something wrong.'*

Everyone has their own way of dealing with stress. How you cope depends partly on the kind of person you are. If you think about how you have handled problems in the past it will give you an idea of how you usually cope.

Some people want to know everything about a problem. They analyse the situation and look for information to try to find a solution. They also seek advice from friends or experts. They buy books like this.

Other people try to ignore the problem. They don't share it with anyone else and they feel that talking about it only makes it worse. This is sometimes called 'denial'. For many people denial is an important and perfectly proper way of dealing with anxiety and fear.

Other things in your life affect how well you can cope. If you have family, job or money worries, or any other difficulties, a health problem may be just one more thing to add to the pile. Or it may be the last straw. And upsetting things in the past which you thought were over and done with, can rear their heads again when you are faced with a new stress.

There is no one way of coping and you must do what is right for you. If you can 'switch off' from the problem and just get on with life, fine. If you are the sort of person who needs to find other people to talk to, do that. Either way, more information may help to get things straight.

Living with the news

'I felt dirty, as if I had something contagious and everyone knew.'

'I really thought I was going to die. I became neurotic, obsessed with my health.'

'I just didn't think about it. I didn't even tell my husband till the day of the hospital appointment.'

If you are being referred to hospital for further examination you may unfortunately have to wait. The services are under a great deal of pressure. Everyone is aware of how distressing the waiting can be, but it is important that all women are treated with equal care and concern.

Even when you are over the initial shock, you probably won't feel back to normal. Illnesses, particularly unusual ones, make most people feel sad and afraid. This can lead to anxiety and depression. You may well have periods of feeling very low or even angry about what is happening to you. This can affect your everyday life and relationships. Some women find it very difficult to concentrate on their jobs or their families with something that feels like a threat hanging over them.

It may particularly affect your relationship with your partner. Many women feel guilty about having a problem 'down below' in the genital area. They feel 'unclean' and are concerned that they may infect their partner, and so they may try to avoid sex. If you feel like this and are unable to tell your partner about it, it can lead to further guilt and resentment on both sides.

Because of the link between sexual activity and cervical cancer, some women also feel very angry and blame their partner or partners. Or they blame themselves, or fear that their partner will, and so feel afraid to discuss the problem. But it is very important that both you and your partner remember that even though sexual contact is involved in the development of most cervical cancers, it doesn't mean either of you has been promiscuous. As explained in Chapter 3, all it needs is one contact by one or other of you, maybe years before you met, to lead to the development of the disease now.

Anger and guilt can put an intolerable strain on any relationship. If you can overcome this enough to talk about your feelings, it can bring a great sense of release. It also makes it easier for other people to help you. Sharing the experience of diagnosis and treatment brings some couples very close together.

If your partner can't give you that kind of support, or you don't have a partner, you may be able to turn to family or friends for help. Or you may find it easier to turn to someone outside – the clinic nurse or counsellor, perhaps. Or you may prefer to work things out for yourself.

Steps to help yourself

'The family still needed looking after. On the surface I played the efficient housewife, and being busy helped. At least it gave me less time to worry.'

'My boyfriend and I played a lot of squash. I took my anger out on the ball. I even started winning!'

'I talked about it endlessly with a friend. I must have got very boring, but she was very patient and it helped.'

Anyone who becomes ill looks back over what they may have done to cause it. It doesn't help. You cannot change what you have done in the past. Try to look forward, because there are things you can do now.

Do whatever helps you to come to terms with the problem, whether it's reading and talking about it, or thinking it over quietly, or taking your mind off it by watching television or going for long runs. Anything – as long as it doesn't harm your health!

You can also try to cut down on smoking or better still, stop.

Women who smoke are much more at risk of cervical cancer. Some women feel easier about intercourse if they use a barrier method of contraception, and it is a sure way to prevent infection being passed between partners.

If you are not being referred to hospital you will need to have follow-up smears. Take your doctor's advice about this. A few women don't attend for further smears or appointments. That may be because they don't get the information, or don't understand why it's necessary, or through fear. It is important to remember that treatment is available and nearly 100% of women with pre-cancer are quickly and simply cured. The investigations don't involve pain and only a minimum of discomfort and indignity. They are described in the next chapter. And remember that sacrificing your dignity is a small price to pay for saving your life.

Chapter 8
The next step – colposcopy

If you have an abnormal smear you will be referred to a gynaecologist – a doctor specialising in the diseases of women. You will receive an appointment for a colposcopy clinic, probably at your local hospital, where you will have further investigations and treatment. This chapter describes what colposcopy is and what it's like to have it done.

What is colposcopy?

A colposcope is a low-power microscope. It doesn't show up individual cells, but it allows the gynaecologist to get the sort of look at the cervix that you can get of the skin with a powerful hand lens. The word comes from the Greek for vagina – *colpos*.

Why do I need colposcopy?

Two reasons: first, to get enough information to plan treatment, and second, to treat you.

As explained in Chapter 4, the smear test collects only scattered cells, and though the cytologist can see if they are abnormal and estimate how severe the dysplasia is, the test doesn't show for certain whether the cells have started invading through the basement membrane. Nor does it give any idea of where round the cervix the dysplasia is. And you can't be treated effectively unless the gynaecologist knows exactly how severe the problem is and exactly where it is.

This information can be gained by colposcopy. An experienced colposcopist (person trained to use a colposcope) can tell by looking closely at the cervix which areas are abnormal and how severely so. It's very important to be totally sure whether or not there is any micro-invasion so the gynaecologist will also take a biopsy, a tiny piece of cervical tissue which will then be processed and examined in a manner similar to the way smears are treated. However, since the biopsy leaves the cells arranged as they were in the body, what the pathologist – the doctor who examines the biopsy – sees down the microscope looks like the diagrams in Chapter 2, so he or she can tell the gynaecologist exactly how far the disease has progressed.

Most women with abnormal smears can be treated by laser, and their treatment is planned and often given using the colposcope. All the different treatments are described in the next chapter.

Shall I have to wait for an appointment?

Unfortunately, the answer is almost always 'yes'. This can be a very worrying time and there is no doubt that in an ideal world there wouldn't be a delay. But even if you do have to wait several weeks the dysplasia changes so very slowly that it won't get worse in that time.

What if I have a period at the time of my appointment?

It's only a problem if your periods are very heavy. Telephone the clinic if you are in doubt.

I do not look forward to going to the clinic

It is an ordeal for everybody. In fact, some women get so worked up that they are too frightened to keep their appointment. They then have the worst of both worlds – knowing that something is wrong, but not having it put right.

Chapter 7 described the reactions many women feel about

having an abnormal smear, and suggested ways of coping with them. You may find it helpful to ask someone to go with you to the clinic. They can give you moral support and also ask questions and listen to what is said when you are too keyed up to be able to do so.

Like some people, you and your partner may decide that he should go with you since it is something that involves the two of you very personally. Or you may feel it is a good reason for taking someone else who is not quite so emotionally involved – perhaps a good friend, someone you trust and can talk to, but not a relative. Some people ask their mothers to come along, though we aren't sure that it is always a good idea – mothers tend to be even more anxious than their daughters and can make you feel less prepared and not more!

We suggest you take with you a list of questions you would like answered. There are some listed at the back of the book. Write your questions down because you won't remember them all while you are there, especially if the staff are very busy and don't give you much time to think.

Most hospitals have a coffee bar. You may find it helps to calm your nerves to sit down and have a cup of coffee before you go to the clinic.

How is a colposcopy clinic organised?

> *'The counsellor talked to us all at once, then people asked questions. I'd have been too embarrassed even on my own to ask about things like sex, so I was glad someone else did.'*
>
> *'I was amazed at how many other women were there. I'd thought I was the only person with an abnormal smear.'*
>
> *'We swapped telephone numbers so we could find out how we'd all got on. It was a great help.'*

Colposcopy clinics vary a lot. This description is based on our clinic. We know that some clinics are much more helpful and supportive than others.

As with any surgery, you are likely to have to wait. There may be a special waiting-room for the clinic, or it may be attached to the general out-patients in which case you won't know what the other people have come for.

If there is a special waiting-room you may well find that someone, probably a special counsellor, will chat to you, either privately or to all the women as a group, or both, about what is going to happen, and possible results, and give you a chance to ask questions. This can be very helpful and many women, though they may at first be put off by finding other people there, gain a great deal of confidence from knowing they aren't the only ones, and from sharing the experience.

When it's your turn, you will be called through to the surgery. There will be a couch, probably in the middle of the room, and the colposcope and other bits and pieces, including probably the doctor's coffee cup – so many women need colposcopy now that the clinics go on for a long time.

If you have brought someone with you to the clinic, she may be asked to wait outside while you are examined. But if it's important to you, ask if she can come in. Either way, she should be allowed to be there when you are given the results.

You may be put off to find there are several people there in addition to the gynaecologist and you. The pathologist may attend the clinic so that he or she can compare the smear and the biopsy with the appearance of the cervix. There will be a nurse who organises the notes and appointments. The counsellor may come in and sit with you. So far, so good. But there may be one or two other people in there who, strictly speaking, aren't essential. They may be local GPs, other gynaecologists, or possibly student doctors, and they have come along to learn about colposcopy. If you really feel you can't go through with it with extra people there, you should mention it and they will leave while you are seen, but do try to remember that the more people who know about colposcopy and can do it, the better the service for women will be in the future.

What is colposcopy like?

'Quite frankly, after several smears, I'd forgotten all about dignity. I was just relieved that something was being done.'

'Apparently some doctors start telling you the result while you're still lying there. I was glad they gave me time to get dressed. It's easier to take in what you're told with your knickers on.'

As with having a smear, because of the inaccessibility of the cervix, it involves some contortions! You will be asked to lie back on the doctor's couch with your bottom at the end and your feet up supported either on foot rests or in stirrups, and your knees flopped open. It isn't very elegant but there's no other way to do the job.

The gynaecologist will then insert a speculum and look down the colposcope at your cervix. Your cervix may be painted with a vinegar-like fluid which makes the areas of dysplasia easier to see. You can't feel it being done. The gynaecologist will then take biopsies – one or maybe several. You may feel a slight twinge while that is being done, but little more. Then the gynaecologist will make a drawing of your cervix in your notes to record what was found. Figure 8/1 shows a typical colposcopy record.

When you are dressed again the gynaecologist will discuss with you what the colposcopy showed. You will probably be feeling very nervous and unable to take it all in, so you may want to ask for your companion to be there. Although the biopsy results won't be available for several days, the gynaecologist will be nearly certain what treatment you will need and will probably make arrangements for you to come back for that, usually very soon. Should the biopsy results show that you need something different from what was expected, you will be informed, possibly by phone or letter or perhaps when you go back to the clinic.

Do ask questions. It is much better to take a little time then than to worry later. And if you think of things after you have left the clinic, you may be able to phone the counsellor or someone else to ask. Don't hesitate to do so.

Fig. 8/1 A typical colposcopy record

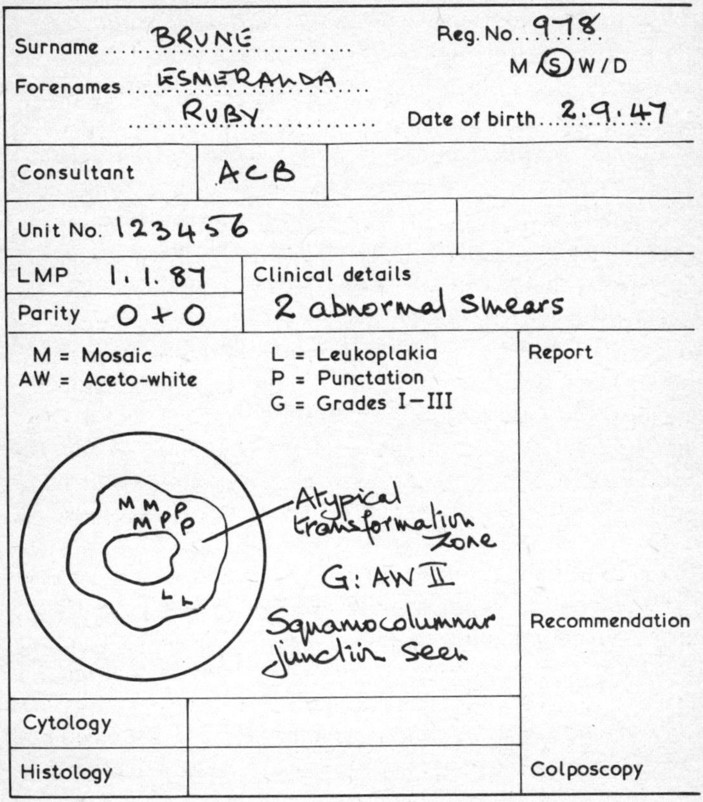
Surname BRUNE
Reg. No. 978
M (S) W/D
Forenames ESMERANDA
RUBY
Date of birth 2.9.47

Consultant ACB

Unit No. 123456

LMP 1.1.87
Parity 0 + 0
Clinical details
2 abnormal smears

M = Mosaic
AW = Aceto-white
L = Leukoplakia
P = Punctation
G = Grades I–III

Report

Recommendation

Cytology

Histology

Colposcopy

Will there be any after-effects from the colposcopy?

> *'He said I'd need laser treatment, but it didn't worry me any more because everyone at the clinic was very kind. It was easier than I'd been imagining.'*

> *'It hadn't hurt, but I felt unclean afterwards, probably because I didn't know what to expect and they didn't explain.'*

The places that were biopsied may bleed a little and it is as well to wait a few days for your cervix to heal before having sex again. Otherwise, there are no physical after-effects. And it is quite safe to have a bath as soon as you want.

How you feel in yourself depends a lot on the clinic and, of course, on the results of your investigation. Unfortunately, at some clinics it is a bit like being on a production line and you may come out of it feeling much the worse for wear. The disease being what it is – the forerunner of cancer – and where it is – 'down there' – some women find the idea of sex very off-putting for a while afterwards, in which case it will help a lot if you can talk to your partner about your experience.

If everything was explained so you knew what was going to happen and what may happen in the future, you will probably feel a sense of relief after your clinic appointment. At least you will have got over the fear of the unknown and know what's going on, which is often the worst part of the battle.

Chapter 9
Treatments

All forms of treatment are designed to do the same thing – to remove or destroy the abnormal cells.

In this chapter we look at the different treatments, when they are used and what it is like to have them.

How may cervical dysplasia and cervical cancer be treated?

Abnormal cells can be destroyed by freezing (*cryocautery*), burning (*diathermy* and *electrocoagulation*) or vaporisation (*laser*). They can be removed by *cone biopsy* or *hysterectomy*. Advanced cancer is unsuitable for either approach and is usually treated by radiotherapy. Each form of treatment has its own advantages and disadvantages.

Who gets which treatment?

This depends principally on how far the disease has progressed, but other factors are important.

Most cases of dysplasia can be treated by destroying the abnormal cells. This can be done on an out-patient basis with laser therapy, cryocautery or low-temperature electrocoagulation (cold coagulation). They can also be done under an anaesthetic. Diathermy cauterisation is painful and needs to be done under anaesthetic.

A cone biopsy is a small operation designed to remove rather than destroy the area of abnormal cervix. Before other treatments became widely available most women with pre-cancer had cone biopsies and it is still necessary in cases where the dysplasia is inaccessible. A cone biopsy will also be recommended on the odd occasion when the gynaecologist feels doubt about what is going on despite colposcopy and biopsy.

Once the abnormal cells have become invasive much more widespread treatment is necessary to be sure that they have all been removed or destroyed. Whether that is by hysterectomy or radiotherapy depends on how far the invading cells have spread, on the facilities available and on the woman's health.

How does laser treatment work?

With laser treatment, abnormal cells can be destroyed simply, quickly, painlessly and economically at one out-patient appointment.

A laser (the letters stand for Light Amplification by Stimulated Emission of Radiation) converts energy from one form into another which can be focused to produce a pinpoint of very intense power. Lasers can be used for many different things as can be seen from pop concerts and James Bond films. The laser used in treating dysplasia is focused on an abnormal area of cervix using the colposcope. It is then switched on and it vaporises the cells in that area. Despite the intense power of the beam it cannot penetrate far and there is no danger of its destroying more than is necessary. Because the abnormal epithelium only is destroyed, the cervix heals perfectly afterwards.

The laser can be used to treat any dysplasia which is visible down the colposcope. The beam can travel only in a straight line so if there is dysplasia round the corner in the cervical canal, a cone biopsy will be needed to remove it. Lasers can also be used for cutting and some gynaecologists use a laser to help to cut a cone biopsy.

Laser treatment has enormous advantages. It is quick and simple for everyone, doctor and patient alike. Most women find it much less of an ordeal than going to the dentist. And it is extremely effective; 95% of women are cured by one treatment.

The only disadvantage is the cost of the equipment – hence the 'Raise a Laser' appeals by many hospitals. We've put a lot of work into 'laser-raising' and we hope that readers of this book will appreciate how worthwhile it is and support – or perhaps launch – appeals in their areas.

What is laser treatment like?

> *'The laser didn't worry me. Everything was explained and it wasn't painful.'*
>
> *'They didn't explain what they were going to do and I felt like a piece of meat in a factory. I felt awful about it for ages.'*
>
> *'I was just relieved because it meant that I wasn't going to get cancer.'*

Laser treatment is usually done at the colposcopy clinic and involves much the same procedure as colposcopy. You, and everyone else in the clinic, will be given unbecoming protective glasses to wear during the procedure, though the risk of damage to the eyes is very small. You may receive an injection of local anaesthetic into your cervix before the treatment. If you are given an injection, you will hardly feel it. If you aren't, don't panic. Even without it, the treatment causes very little pain – much less than having a tooth filled.

The gynaecologist will then identify the areas of dysplasia and laser them. It takes about ten minutes. You may feel some mild discomfort but rarely anything more. There may be a slight smell of burning as the laser does its work. If the clinic has closed-circuit television you can watch it on that – if you want to!

After the treatment you may have some mild pain for a few hours, in which case it is quite safe to take aspirin or paracetamol, or whatever you prefer, to ease it. Some clinics suggest you take two paracetamol tablets just before your appointment just in case.

The most unpleasant after-effect of laser treatment is the messy and blood-stained discharge which may last for a couple of weeks. It is the destroyed tissue coming away, together with some bleeding from the raw area. A nuisance, but normal as long as you aren't losing more than a period.

For two weeks, or until the discharge stops (in other words until the cervix is healing over), you should not put anything in the vagina because of the risk of infection. Use sanitary pads rather than tampons and avoid having intercourse.

After the discharge has stopped you can use tampons again and it is safe to resume love-making. But the cervix is still fragile and your partner should use a sheath for the next two months to protect it, in addition to whatever method of contraception you are using.

The treatment doesn't directly affect your periods, though some people find that worry affects their cycles so your next period may be a bit early or a bit late.

What happens after I have had laser treatment?

You will need a follow-up examination in a few months to check that your cervix has healed. One laser treatment cures almost everyone, so you can get on with the rest of your life – and that includes getting pregnant if you wish – with confidence. But like every other woman, it is still possible that you may develop dysplasia in the future, so you will still need regular smear tests. For a while, the gynaecologist will want to keep a particularly close eye on your cervix, so you will be asked to have a smear every year. That can be a reminder of things you would prefer to put out of your mind, but remember, you have been cured and whatever the smears may show, you are not going to get cancer.

What is cryocautery?

'The messy discharge afterwards was a nuisance.'

'My husband wasn't too impressed when I told him we couldn't have sex for a few weeks but we coped.'

Cryocautery is destruction of abnormal cells by freezing them –

cryo is Greek for cold. You may have had warts on the hands treated this way. Like laser treatment, it can be done in the clinic.

Having cryocautery is similar to having laser treatment, although it takes longer. Its advantage is that the equipment is cheaper and more widely available and there are gynaecologists who are not trained to use a laser but who can perform cryocautery, so if you live a long way from a clinic with a laser you may have cryocautery instead. It has two main disadvantages. It does more damage to the cervix, although it is most unlikely that you would have trouble in pregnancy and labour in the future. Also, the cure rate is often not quite so high as with laser treatment, so it is particularly important that you have regular smear tests after cryocautery.

What is electrocautery or diathermy?

Heat as well as cold can destroy tissue. Some forms of heat cautery can be done on an out-patient basis in a clinic, but most require a day in hospital and a general anaesthetic because they are painful. Electrocautery, also called diathermy, is a very effective treatment for dysplasia. It's as neat and efficient as laser treatment without the need for special equipment and training.

What is a cone biopsy?

A cone biopsy is the removal of a cone-shaped piece of the cervix including the transformation zone and part of the canal. Figure 9/1 shows what is removed and why it is called a *cone* biopsy.

If you need a cone biopsy it does not mean you have more serious disease. It means that the gynaecologist cannot be sure that other treatments will remove all the abnormal cells.

If the area of dysplasia disappears up the cervical canal the laser won't touch it because the beam cannot go round corners. And if the preceding investigations have shown adenocarcinoma the abnormal tissue is again out of range in the cervical

Fig. 9/1 A cone biopsy

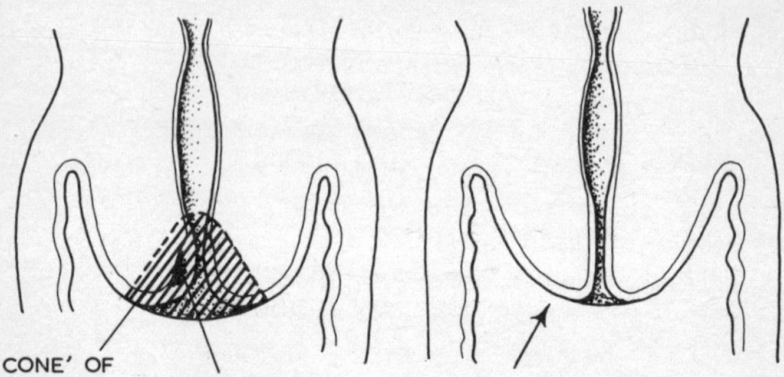

canal. So it is necessary to do a cone biopsy, because it removes the area the laser cannot reach.

A cone biopsy may be done because the gynaecologist isn't sure what is going on. Sometimes the biopsy taken at colposcopy isn't adequate – like anything, it is impossible to do it perfectly every time. Sometimes the findings from the smear, the colposcopy appearance of the cervix and the biopsies suggest different things, so a cone biopsy is done to make certain.

Cone biopsies are called biopsies because they are a way of getting tissue so that it can be examined by the pathologist. They permit a diagnosis to be made. At the same time they can be curative because the abnormal tissue is removed. It is most important that the pathologist examines the edges of the biopsy. As long as there is normal tissue at the edges, and no sign of invasion anywhere, no further treatment is needed.

What is it like to have a cone biopsy?

'I was very apprehensive and I had to stay in hospital an extra day because I couldn't pee – probably because I'd worked myself up into a state. It wasn't necessary because it was no worse than having my wisdom teeth out, but it's easy to say that after the event.'

'One thing about going into hospital, you realise how many people are worse off than yourself.'

'I bled quite a lot afterwards and was worried until I rang up and they reassured me that it was normal.'

You will probably be admitted to hospital the day before your biopsy. The operation requires a general anaesthetic and it takes about fifteen minutes. When the cone has been removed the surgeon will put a few dissolvable stitches in your cervix and may pack your vagina with gauze to stop the bleeding. The pack will be removed the next day. Occasionally women have difficulty passing water after the operation and need a catheter – a tube in the bladder to drain the urine – overnight until they can get going again. All being well you will be home in a day or two.

Some hospitals are experimenting with admitting women for cone biopsy just for one day. A general anaesthetic may still be required but the biopsy is cut using a laser which reduces the risk of bleeding.

After the operation you will need to take it easy for a week or two, as your cervix needs all your energy to heal. Pain isn't usually a problem, but bleeding may be. You are bound to lose some blood from the raw area and this may be quite heavy, especially about a week after the operation. You need only contact a doctor if you are in severe pain, or if the bleeding is heavier than a period and doesn't stop, or if you have a smelly discharge. As with laser treatment you should use pads rather than tampons and, because the cervix has a lot more healing to do, avoid sex for at least a month and use sheaths for a while when you resume intercourse.

What happens after a cone biopsy?

'I've had a baby since my cone biopsy, and there were no problems, I'm glad to say.'

You will be given an appointment for the clinic when the doctor will check that your cervix is healing and discuss the pathologist's report with you. Assuming you need no further treatment you will then go back to regular smear checks, like women who have had laser treatment.

Once your cervix has healed, the cone biopsy will make no difference to either you or your partner when you have sex.

Because cone biopsy takes quite a bite out of the cervix, it doesn't heal as neatly as a lasered or cauterised cervix. It is most unlikely to stop you getting pregnant, but it can sometimes lead to early labour. The labour itself is usually perfectly normal. You should certainly tell the people looking after you in your pregnancy that you have had a cone biopsy, but there is no need to worry about getting pregnant on that account.

When is hysterectomy needed?

Hysterectomy, the removal of the uterus, is a much bigger procedure.

It is very rarely done in cases of dysplasia because it isn't necessary. Simpler treatments are perfectly adequate. If someone with dysplasia has a hysterectomy there are generally other reasons. For instance, a woman who has completed her family and is having severe problems with heavy bleeding, who then finds she has dysplasia may decide that a hysterectomy would kill two birds with one stone. No more periods and no dysplasia. Even though the cervix is competely removed in the operation, you will need follow-up smears to check that the vagina is not affected by the disease.

A hysterectomy may also become necessary when there is true cancer. If a cancer is micro-invasive – discovered on biopsy but otherwise undetectable – or if it is big enough to have caused bleeding and to be visible on examination, but still confined to the cervix, a hysterectomy can often completely cure because the surgeon removes the whole cervix with the tumour, plus enough tissue from round it to 'catch' any cells that have escaped. In cases of more advanced cancer where the tumour has spread beyond the cervix, hysterectomy may still be recommended to remove the bulk of the cancer but it is unlikely to be sufficient.

Hysterectomy is a big subject and so it is considered fully in the next chapter.

What is radiotherapy and when is it needed?

A very short exposure to a very low dose of *x*-rays can be used to make a picture of the body – the familiar *x*-ray. Most people know that too many *x*-rays have the potential to harm the body. That potential can be put to good use by using *x*-rays, in a large dose, to destroy cancer cells. Radiotherapy is usually given as a course of short out-patient sessions over several days or weeks.

Radiotherapy itself doesn't hurt, though some people feel slightly nauseated or develop a headache during treatment. There are usually side-effects afterwards, such as diarrhoea or cystitis (symptoms like having a urine infection) which can be troublesome, but they usually settle once the course of treatment is finished. Radiotherapy to the cervix inevitably affects the ovaries and leads to sterility. Since that is irreversible, it means the end of childbearing.

Radiotherapy is only used for true cancer. It can destroy abnormal cells scattered over a wide area and so is usually the treatment recommended for those whose cancer has spread beyond the cervix. But it is also effective for early cancers, and in those cases it saves a major operation, an advantage for a woman who is too unwell for surgery or perhaps for someone who hates the idea of it.

Whatever method of treatment is recommended to you, the pros and cons should be explained to you. Even the worst experiences are much less alarming if you know what to expect. If you don't understand, or are worried, *ask*.

Chapter 10
Hysterectomy

Most women who have an abnormal smear can be cured with simple out-patient treatment, as described in the previous chapter. Only a few women will need a hysterectomy. But a hysterectomy is much more of an ordeal, so we have devoted a chapter to it.

Why do women need a hysterectomy?

As outlined in Chapter 9, there are two main reasons for the gynaecologist to recommend a hysterectomy.

The first is for true cancer. Once cells have become malignant and broken through the basement membrane, destroying them by laser or cautery is not enough. As long as the cancer is confined to the cervix, hysterectomy – removal of the whole uterus including the cervix – can cure the disease.

The second is for pre-cancers associated with other problems. These include heavy or frequent periods and fibroids. If a woman does not want children or has completed her family, then hysterectomy may be suggested.

Is the operation the same for everyone?

No. The way the operation is performed and how much is removed will vary according to need.

If the operation is required for true cancer what is called a

Wertheim's hysterectomy is performed. The whole uterus, a small part of the top of the vagina, and the tissue around the uterus containing lymph nodes (glands) are removed. If a woman has not yet gone through the menopause, the surgeon will probably leave her ovaries.

If a hysterectomy is performed for a woman who has pre-cancer there is no need to take so much because the abnormal cells have not escaped from the basement membrane. Only the uterus is removed, and in a woman past the menopause, the ovaries.

A hysterectomy for cervical cancer is usually done through a cut in the abdomen. Occasionally, if the woman is also suffering from prolapse, and as long as she only has pre-cancer, the operation may be done from down below via the vagina. In that case a cut in the abdomen is not needed.

Removal of the uterus means an end to childbearing and an end to periods. However, if your ovaries are left behind you will still be aware of other aspects of your monthly cycle – pre-menstrual symptoms for example, because these are caused by the female hormones released by the ovaries. And in time you may experience the symptoms of the menopause – hot flushes, night sweats and vaginal dryness for instance, even though your periods stopped when you had the operation maybe many years before. If your ovaries are removed along with your uterus while you are still having periods, you will start experiencing menopausal symptoms quite soon after the operation. Under these circumstances the symptoms can be quite severe and, especially if you are still quite young, you may be helped by Hormone Replacement Therapy (HRT). However, HRT is not suitable for everyone.

How long will it take to recover?

'I was amazed at how well I felt when I left hospital (after a week).'

'I felt fine when I got up in the mornings, but even making the bed exhausted me at first.'

> *'I didn't feel I could face a classful of 11-year-olds for at least two months.'*

You will be in hospital for between five and fourteen days. This varies from doctor to doctor, and on your general recovery.

No one can predict when you will be back to full fitness. Most women who have had a hysterectomy would agree that it takes between six and twelve weeks and sometimes even longer to feel really on top of things.

You will be up and around and feeling quite well by the time you leave hospital, but when you get home you will need to rest as you will find that you tire quickly. The smallest task can be exhausting. This will improve gradually.

In the first few weeks you may get some aches and pains which can be worrying, but they are quite normal unless they are very severe and prolonged, in which case you should see your doctor. Some vaginal loss, either bright red blood or brown discharge, is also to be expected. Some women have bladder problems, particularly frequency or lack of control. They generally improve with time. The hospital physiotherapist may be able to suggest exercises to help you.

You will be asked to return to hospital for an out-patient check-up appointment about six weeks after the operation. Until then, you should not go back to work or do heavy household chores or anything that requires lifting or stretching. If family or friends cannot give enough assistance, the social services department will provide a home help for a while. You should not drive because you might have trouble braking in an emergency, and you will probably find long journeys as a passenger uncomfortable.

If you have any worries about your recovery, make a list of questions and take them to your appointment. Even if it seems silly or trivial, do ask. If it worries you, it is important.

If all is well at your six-week check, you can gradually increase your activity. You can return to work unless your job is very physically demanding, and you can drive again.

What about sex after a hysterectomy?

Once you are fully healed inside, and that can take three months, neither you or your partner should experience any change as a result of your operation, even if you had the more extensive Wertheim's hysterectomy.

You should resume sexual intercourse when you feel ready, although we suggest that you try at least once, very gently, before your six-week check so that you can let the doctor know if there is a problem. You may feel tense and anxious at first, especially if, like some women, you feel that hysterectomy may have damaged your femininity, and that can make it difficult to enjoy intercourse again until you have got your confidence back. Try to talk it over with your partner so that he can understand how you feel. If you can't talk to him, it may help you to relax if you can discuss it with someone else.

Are there psychological after-effects?

'I just felt relieved that all the worrying was over.'

'I thought I would never feel a proper woman again.'

It is often thought that all the psychological effects of hysterectomy are bad. That is not so. If you have experienced a great deal of anxiety or debilitating long heavy periods you may feel a new sense of well-being and relief that the problem has been solved. Some women find themselves more relaxed because hysterectomy means the end to worries about contraception.

Many women feel a general sense of being 'down' after hysterectomy. The anxiety of illness and going into hospital, tiredness and its limitations on activities all take their toll. These generally pass quite quickly if you take every day as it comes, accepting what you can do today and hoping to do a little more tomorrow.

Unfortunately, some women do feel more seriously emotionally affected by the operation. Knowing you can no longer have children can be a crushing blow. Even if they didn't intend to have any more, the lack of choice and the lack of a womb can make some women feel bereaved, worthless and unfeminine. But femaleness is more than the ability to conceive; it encompasses many aspects of a woman's nature. Women are female before they can conceive and will be female in old age. Several film stars who are bywords for femininity and sex appeal have had hysterectomies.

Where can I get help?

> *'After a lot of dithering I rang up the local Hysterectomy Group and immediately wished I'd had the courage to do it earlier. They put my mind at rest over lots of things, and I stopped feeling so alone. By now I've got my health and my confidence back.'*

> *'My mother told me everyone who had their womb out gets fat like a neutered cat. I was very relieved to find out that's not true.'*

The few pieces of research that have been done show that women appear to recover better after hysterectomy, physically and emotionally, if they have good information before the operation.

Try to find out as much as possible from your doctor. Take a list of questions with you, or ask a relative or friend to accompany you.

If you have problems afterwards, try your GP or practice nurse, or a Well Woman Clinic if you have one near you, or a Family Planning Clinic may be prepared to help. You might also like to contact the Hysterectomy Support Group, whose address is at the back of the book. They will give you straightforward information and put you in touch with other women in your area who have had hysterectomies. Sharing experiences and talking over problems can be very helpful and supportive.

Chapter 11
Advanced cervical cancer

If you are having a smear test, or have had an abnormal result, and have turned to this chapter to discover the worst, you can be reassured. The very fact that you have had a smear test is a good guarantee that you will never develop cervical cancer.

Remember that the smear test detects dysplasia and nearly 100% of women who develop dysplasia are cured. The majority of women who are found to have invasive cancer at an early stage are also cured. So they will not go on to develop advanced cancer.

Unfortunately, every year about 2000 women, most of whom have not had smear tests, do suffer and die from advanced disease. This chapter is about their problems.

What happens as the disease progresses?

Pre-cancer and early true cancer, when the growth is confined to the cervix, are like the newly sprouting weed – both are quite easy to get rid of and not likely to grow back. But if it is left, the weed gets stronger and stronger. It becomes difficult to remove without making a mess of the garden around it. It interferes with the growth of nearby plants. Even if you think you have pulled it all up it may grow back from bits of root left behind, and you can never be sure that it won't sprout up somewhere else from its seeds. Advanced cancer is exactly like the weed.

The progressive growth of cervical cancer is described in

Stages. *Stage 0* is pre-cancer. *Stage I* is cancer confined to the cervix. *Stage II* cancer has grown out of the cervix into the tissues around, but not far. A cancer is *Stage III* if it has spread as far as the lower part of the vagina or the sides of the pelvis, and *Stage IV* if it has invaded the bladder or the back passage, or spread out around the body, for instance to the lungs.

What are the symptoms of advanced cancer?

The cancer forms a lump on the cervix which bleeds easily. It usually becomes infected, causing a smelly discharge. Both are likely to get worse with time. There is rarely any pain until the cancer has spread to *Stage III* or *IV* but then it can become severe. If the bladder and the bowel are affected, there can be blood in the urine, incontinence and bowel problems.

The symptoms are the same as a lot of very minor problems so it's always important to go to the doctor to get them sorted out. Women who are worried that they may have cancer will probably find that their mind is put at rest, but a simple examination will show if there is something seriously wrong and on the rare occasion that happens, the earlier it is found the more can be done.

How is advanced cancer treated?

In the earlier stages of the cancer, some people are always cured, but the number gets fewer as the disease progresses. Doctors will always do their best to cure a patient, but when cancer is very advanced that generally becomes unrealistic.

When the treatment becomes so unpleasant that it is more than a patient can bear, she may request that her doctors stop trying to find a cure and concentrate on simple ways of easing her suffering. The patient always has the choice about this. But for *Stages II* and *III* cancers at least, curing the disease and stopping the symptoms both involve the same thing – destroying the cancer cells. So one form of treatment does both.

By the time cervical cancer has become advanced, that is at least *Stage III*, it is very difficult to do a hysterectomy because the uterus becomes stuck to everything else. Most women will therefore have radiotherapy to destroy the cancer cells. This is likely to be broadly similar to that used for treating the less advanced disease and described in Chapter 9. If you are already feeling unwell the side-effects can be particularly distressing, but they still usually settle down.

Other forms of treatment may be used occasionally. Drug treatment – chemotherapy – usually has very unpleasant side-effects while it is being given, but it can be very effective at shrinking the cancer. And surgeons may sometimes operate to take away much more than just the uterus. This is a big operation and it would never be done without the patient's knowing exactly what it would involve, but for the few people who are suitable it can mean a longer life and better one.

What are the effects of the treatment?

Women being treated for advanced cancer have to cope with a double burden. They have the knowledge that they may die prematurely as well as the physical side-effects of the treatment.

The debilitating effects of radiotherapy and chemotherapy may leave a woman feeling weak, apathetic and without hope. Losing control over what is happening to your body can be depressing and frightening.

How can I cope with the disease and the treatment?

It seems that the more a patient can be involved in her treatment, the more she feels in control, and research has shown that any help given to cancer patients, whether it is sophisticated counselling or simple practical support, reduces anxiety and fear. Knowing what is happening, and why, makes you feel more positive about the outcome. Ask your doctor to explain the treatment and its possible side-effects. Accept all offers of assistance that may make your life easier or more comfortable.

There is nothing wrong with feeling angry or frightened or with expressing those feelings. It can help to talk about how you feel, not just to reduce your anxiety, but also to give those close to you an opportunity to offer help and support.

It is never easy to live with advanced cancer, but the symptoms should be controllable and as long as all hope is not lost, it is possible to make the most of a shortened life span.

Chapter 12
Men and cervical cancer

Cervical cancer is a sexually transmitted disease. Only women can get cervical cancer, but they get it because of their sexual relationships with men. In this chapter we look at the role of men in cervical cancer.

Why are men involved in causing cervical cancer?

As explained in Chapter 3, to develop cervical cancer it is necessary to have been infected by the wart virus, HPV. Women carry the virus on the cervix and men carry it on the penis. And the only way that the virus can be picked up is through having sex with an infected person.

The more partners a woman has, the more likely she is to encounter a man with HPV and so pick up the infection. The more partners a man has, the more likely he is to encounter a woman with HPV and so pick up the infection. But it only requires one exposure to the virus to catch it, and it only requires one sexual experience to pass it on. A couple can be perfectly faithful to each other but if either of them, at any time, possibly long before they met, has just once had sex with an infected person, the woman will be at risk. So neither you nor your partner needs to be at all promiscuous to have HPV infection.

What can men do about it?

Three things: ensure that they do not pick up the infection; ensure that it is treated; and ensure that they do not pass it on.

The first of these is easier said than done. It's easy to condemn sexual freedom but it has brought benefits as well as disadvantages and it's probably here to stay. At the same time cervical cancer, AIDS, and herpes are good reasons for all of us to think that little bit longer before embarking on a new sexual relationship.

Once you have got HPV infection, and a lot of people already have, it seems sensible to try to get rid of it. This is discussed more fully in the next section, but, briefly, HPV doesn't always cause visible warts and it is not easy to be sure that it has been eliminated.

That makes the third thing, making sure that the infection is not passed on, vital – literally. If you are going to have sex and may be infected, you *must* make sure that you have safe sex. And that means the sheath.

The sheath has been out of favour since the advent of the Pill. But 20 years ago we did not have AIDS, we did not have herpes and we did not know about HPV. Now it has overwhelming advantages. Properly used, and with a spermicide, the sheath protects against infection. The virus cannot pass through the sheath, and any that do escape may be killed by the spermicide (it isn't enough to use a spermicide alone, though).

It is vital that men take responsibility for their partner's health by using the sheath every time they make love. And it is up to women to protect their own health by ensuring that their partners have sheaths – by providing them if necessary – *and that they use them and use them properly*.

At present the advertising of sheaths is very restricted. We hope this will change, and that they will become much easier to obtain. It is also essential that all men, and particularly young men, appreciate why a sheath is so important, can get hold of one and feel a responsibility to use it.

We all, as individuals and a society, have to develop new attitudes to sexual activity, and to develop them quickly.

Conditions are changing and we require new notions of responsible sex. Our health depends on it.

What about men with HPV?

'It's not the sort of thing you can talk over with your mates – I could talk about my wife, but not about me.'

We wish we could give definite advice to men about HPV infection. Unfortunately it isn't at all clear what men should be doing.

Certainly, anyone who has warts should be treated. They tend to grow under the foreskin, so uncircumcised men should retract their foreskin to look. Warts can be too small to be seen easily, and ideally we feel that every partner, past and present, of a woman who has an abnormal smear, should be professionally checked for warts.

The place to go for investigation and treatment is the Special Clinic, otherwise known as Department of Genito-urinary Medicine. All clinics will treat warts, but at this stage few clinics offer treatment to men with no visible warts. It is a very new problem for clinics already overloaded with work and people are only just deciding what is the best policy.

Special Clinics are to be found attached to most big hospitals. The details of times and place can be obtained by telephoning the clinic (try the classified section of the telephone directory for the number) or the Family Planning Association will give you the information (see page 83 for the address). Or you can find out from the hospital, your GP, the public library or that traditional source, advertisements in public toilets. You don't need a referral from another doctor, but if you don't make an appointment you will probably have to wait.

You will be examined carefully for warts. Warts will be destroyed or removed. The various treatments are not painful.

Special Clinics undertake 'contact tracing' and since your sexual partners may be infected it is important for their health that you should co-operate with this exercise. The counsellors who do this job are aware of how delicate matters can be and are very discreet.

The problem is that HPV may infect areas that are very difficult to reach – inside the meatus (urinary canal) for example. And even if the penis appears to be clear of infection, either with or without treatment, it seems that it may still be around. So it is very difficult to guarantee that any man is free of it.

So what is the point of seeking treatment? A good question. But if your warts are treated, you will certainly be less infective than untreated. And we hope that the whole matter will become clearer soon.

Does HPV cause cancer in men?

It's possible, but not at all certain, that HPV may slightly increase the risk of cancer of the penis, but that is a very rare disease.

What should a man do if his partner has an abnormal smear?

'I couldn't tell my husband, I thought he'd think I'd been sleeping around.'

'I wanted to help my wife but I thought she was blaming me for giving it to her.'

The most important thing is to give support. Understand that she is likely to be worried about cancer, upset about having a sexually transmitted disease, and apprehensive about the forthcoming treatment. She will be concerned about how it affects her relationship with you. You too will be worried and concerned and it is very important that you help each other.

It can be tempting to wonder who first caught the infection, and when, and from whom. It isn't very helpful – you cannot undo the past and in any case you will probably never know. It is important to put the past behind you and look to the future. Get treatment if you have warts, go with your partner to the colposcopy clinic if she would like you to, and don't be afraid to ask questions on your own account and on hers. As discussed in Chapter 7, knowing they have the disease can make some women very reluctant about sex, which can be particularly stressful. Use a sheath when you do make love, until her cervix has healed after treatment.

It can be a very testing time for couples, but with effort and understanding it can bring you even closer together.

To summarise, the way things are at present there is only one way to live healthily with HPV. That is through safe responsible sex. And for that the sheath is vital.

Chapter 13
Preventing cervical cancer

It is good to be able to cure a disease, but much better to be able to prevent it. Ways of preventing cervical cancer have been mentioned in several of the previous chapters. In this chapter we concentrate on this very important topic.

Cervical cancer can be prevented at two stages of its development: *before* there are any cell changes and *after* dysplasia has developed but while the disease is at the pre-cancerous stage. To prevent women from developing dysplasia they have to be protected from factors which make them susceptible to the disease. To prevent those who have developed dysplasia progressing to true cancer, the dysplasia has to be detected and treated.

How can the development of dysplasia be prevented?

In Chapter 3 we discussed the factors which put women at higher risk of developing cervical cancer. Factors which certainly increase risk are: infection with the human papilloma or wart virus, sexual activity, smoking and taking the Pill. In addition, pregnancy may increase the risk, and it is likely that in time it will become clear that there are other risk factors.

Not everyone who gets infected with cervical wart virus develops dysplasia, but it seems that every woman with dysplasia has at some time had wart virus infection and that the infection is in some way essential to trigger the development of the disease. Therefore, if no one got the infection no one would get cervical cancer (at least, not the common squamous carcinoma). How can this be achieved?

In theory the virus could be eliminated from the world. This has been done with the smallpox virus by vaccinating everyone against it. Unfortunately there is no vaccine against HPV – yet. As yet not enough is known about the virus – its link with cervical cancer has only become clear in the last few years – but researchers are working on it. There is no doubt that when it can be done, vaccination provides the most logical and practical way to eliminate the disease entirely.

Until a vaccine has been developed, tested, and proved to be safe, and that may take many years, the best we can do is to prevent women from becoming infected by HPV. Since it is spread by sexual activity, as explained in Chapter 3, that means a change in sexual habits. The fewer sexual partners any person, male or female, has, the lower their risk of picking up the virus and so the lower the risk of the woman in any partnership becoming infected. So in theory absolute chastity would eliminate the spread; not a very realistic proposition. In any case, it only requires one sexual contact to pick up the virus. Furthermore, unless they have had a recent smear test women have no means of knowing that they have HPV, and nor have men unless they have visible warts. So anyone who has ever had any sexual contact may potentially be a carrier.

The realistic answer to risky sex is safe sex – in other words, the sheath and a spermicide. The combination provides very good protection against infection with HPV. Other barrier methods of contraception such as the diaphragm (Dutch Cap) are much less effective against infection because they allow much more contact between the penis and the vagina, and although the spermicide which is used with them helps because it can kill the virus, it is not 100% efficient.

The use of the sheath is discussed more fully in Chapter 12, so just to recap – prevention of cervical cancer by prevention of spread of the wart virus depends on use of the sheath and spermicide in all sexual relations outside stable monogamous partnerships. That is a lot to ask, but the price of failing is likely to be much illness and unhappiness.

As for the other risk factors, as described in Chapter 3, smoking increases the chances of developing dysplasia quite significantly; taking the Pill and pregnancy much less so. An individual woman can reduce her risk by stopping smoking, but even if everyone gave up smoking today, some women would still develop the disease. And it is hardly practical to eliminate the last risk factor mentioned – pregnancy!

There is a further problem, and that is adenocarcinoma. This is the less common form of cervical cancer, and as discussed in Chapter 4, as far as we know at present, none of the risk factors for the more common squamous carcinoma leads to adenocarcinoma. Since we do not know what causes it, we are not in a position to protect people and so to prevent it.

To summarise, at present, and being realistic, we cannot prevent cervical cancer. But a change in sexual habits, especially by use of the sheath, and a reduction in smoking, would reduce the numbers of women who develop the disease quite considerably.

How can true cancer be prevented?

By smear tests to detect pre-cancer and then treatment to destroy or remove the abnormal cells. If all women were effectively screened, no one need die from cervical cancer.

We cannot stop women developing pre-cancer but we can prevent them suffering severe consequences. The tragedy is that ignorance of the true facts, or misunderstanding of them, or embarrassment, or inadequate facilities, or haphazard administrative arrangements, or outdated medical priorities all play a part in 2000 preventable deaths a year.

Chapter 14
The future

It will be obvious from the preceding chapters that a great deal remains to be understood about cervical cancer. What is clear is that the disease is changing and it is on the increase, especially among young women. All the more important, then, that we find out more about it so we are in a better position to prevent it, to detect it and to treat it. In this chapter we look at likely future developments.

Understanding the disease

With careful collection of statistics, and comparisons of women who develop the disease with women who do not, and studies of the way the disease behaves in individual cases, we have begun to learn about why it happens and how it develops. It is this sort of work that has shown the role played by the wart virus in triggering the disease, and has led to the identification of other risk factors. It has also demonstrated the progression from normal cells through dysplasia to true cancer. Eventually – these studies take a long time – we shall understand cervical cancer much better, and that is essential if we are to prevent and cure it.

Preventing the disease

Ultimately, we can hope to have a vaccine to prevent cervical cancer, but development and testing will take many years. Until then, our best course lies in preventing the spread of the wart virus. It may become possible to treat men so they can be sure they don't carry the virus. In the immediate future, safety from cervical cancer lies in responsible sex. The use of the sheath to prevent disease was a Victorian habit which went out when antibiotics were discovered, but now it is due for a comeback. It is to be hoped that with education and encouragement aimed specially at young people sex can be made safer.

Detecting pre-cancer

The system for smear testing in this country is in the process of reorganisation so in the future fewer women should slip through the net. There are also developments in smear-testing technique to make the test easier to take, so that there are fewer inadequate smears, and easier to analyse so that less time and effort are needed in the laboratory. This work involves using the techniques of genetic engineering to identify special chemicals present only in dysplastic cells. Maybe in time a smear will not be necessary and all that will be needed will be a blood test.

Curing pre-cancer

In the immediate future the most important thing is the spread of facilities for colposcopy and treatment of dysplasia. The more clinics there are – and that means the more doctors are trained and the more colposcopes that are available – the better the service to women.

Curing and coping with cancer

A diagnosis of cancer used to be like a death knell. That is not necessarily so any more, and every year the list of curable cancers grows. Cervical cancer is a cancer that can actually be prevented, and if it does develop, cured in many cases.

Many of the people who do develop cervical cancer do so

because they are frightened of it and so don't take advantage of smear testing. In the future, more and more people will realise, because of personal experience or more information, that cancer can often be cured especially if it's caught early. Such a change in attitude to cancer will encourage more women to have smear tests and will help those who develop the disease to come to terms with it. And with time, our ability to treat true cancer will improve so there will be less to fear.

Women are increasingly taking action themselves to improve their health care facilities. Much of the impetus for Well Woman Clinics has come from small groups of women who saw there was a need for clinics in their areas and campaigned to set them up. The Women's National Cancer Control Campaign has done a great deal not only to spread information and stimulate national interest but also to provide mobile smear-testing facilities. Some trade unions and private companies are taking positive steps to encourage women to have smears by using mobile units and allowing women to attend in working hours.

Self-help groups have been started for women with cancer by women with personal experience of the disease. They are able to offer information and support and to provide an invaluable supplement to the work of the health care professionals.

Things get done because people know about them and think they are important. If we talk about cervical cancer now, and even shout about it when necessary, we can make sure that in the future it becomes a disease of the past.

Glossary

adenocarcinoma Rare form of cervical cancer

biopsy Small piece of tissue removed for laboratory examination for the purpose of making a diagnosis

cervix Neck of the uterus (womb)

CIN Cervical intraepithelial neoplasia: the term used in grading pre-cancerous changes of the cervix

colposcopy A method of examining the surface of the cervix

cone biopsy A cone-shaped piece of the cervix removed under general anaesthetic for laboratory examination

cryocautery Freezing technique used to destroy abnormal parts of the cervix

dyskariosis The word used to describe abnormal cells seen when reporting on a smear

dysplasia Development of abnormal cells

ectropion Appearance of the cervix when there are columnar cells on the visible part of the cervix

epithelium Surface layer of a tissue

erosion Common term for an ectropion

HPV Human Papilloma Virus

koilocytes Type of cells seen when there is HPV infection

laser Highly focused beam of light capable of destroying abnormal cells by vaporising them

Papanicolaou First described the technique of cervical smear: hence the term 'Pap smear'

smear Scraping of cells from the cervix examined under a microscope to identify any abnormal cells

speculum An instrument passed into the vagina to display the cervix

wart virus See Human Papilloma Virus (HPV)

Questions to ask your doctor

These are some of the questions you may want to ask the doctor. At times of stress remembering all these questions may not be easy so we suggest you write down some of these and any others you think of.

Having the smear

When will the results be available?
How shall I be notified of the result?
Is it necessary for me to phone if I do not have the result by the time you say I shall?

The results

Normal
When should I have another smear?
Will I be called for the smear or do I have to arrange it myself?
If I have to arrange it myself, whom do I contact?
Abnormal
What is the abnormality?
What does it mean to me?
What is the next step?
How shall I be notified?

Colposcopy

What are the findings at the time of colposcopy?
If a biopsy has been done, when will the results be available and who will tell me?
What treatment shall I have to have, and when will it be done?

Treatment

What does the treatment involve?
- is an anaesthetic needed?
- shall I need to stay in hospital?

May I bring along a friend or partner?
Do I need to bring anything with me (e.g. sanitary towel)?
What are the follow-up arrangements?

Questions of your own

Useful organisations

Addresses and telephone numbers given are those of the head office of each organisation. Where local organisations exist, the best method of contacting them is indicated.

Bacup
121–3 Charterhouse Street
London EC1 M6AA 01 608 1661
Cancer information service staffed by trained nurses to give general and medical advice to cancer patients and their families.

Brook Advisory Centres
153A East Street
London SE17 01 708 1234
Birth-control clinics, but dealing with all problems relating to sex and sex-linked diseases. Some branches specialise in information and help for young people. Local centres are listed in telephone directory.

Cancerlink
46 Pentonville Road
London N1 01 833 2451
Information and support for people with cancer and their families and friends. Details of local branches from head office.

Community Health Council See local Telephone Directory
Councils exist in most cities and will give information about any health-related topic, including:

Where to get a smear test
Well Woman Clinics
Family Planning Clinics

Family Planning Association
27–35 Mortimer Street
London W1 01 636 7866

Family Planning Information Service
27 St Peter's Street
Bedford MK40 2PN 0234 62436
13A Western Road
Hove BN3 1AE 0273 774075
4 Barnfield Hill
Exeter EX1 1SR 0392 56711
6 Windsor Place
Cardiff CF1 3BX 0222 42766
20A Bridewell Alley
Norwich NR2 1SY 0603 628704
5 York Road
Birmingham B16 9HX 021 454 8236
9 Gambier Terrace
Liverpool L1 7BQ 051 709 1938
17 North Church Street
Sheffield S1 2DH 0742 21191
4 Clifton Street
Glasgow G3 7LA 041 333 9696
160 Shepherd's Bush Road
London W6 7PB 01 602 2723
113 University Street
Belfast BT7 1HP 0232 225488
Information, including leaflets, posters and publications, and enquiry service on all aspects of family planning, personal relationships and sex-related diseases.

Healthcall 0898 600 600
Healthline (College of Health) 01 980 4848
Information services providing tapes on many topics, including cervical cancer.

Hysterectomy Support Groups
11 Henryson Road
London SE4 01 690 5987
Advice, information and support for women having a hysterectomy. Details of local groups available from head office.

WHIC – Women's Health Information Centre
52 Featherstone Street
London EC1 01 251 6580
Open weekdays 12–4pm, Wednesdays 2–6pm.
Information and support on a wide range of women's health problems.

Women's National Cancer Control Campaign
1 South Audley Street
London W1 01 499 7532
Information, campaigning, mobile smear testing.

Women's Health Concern
17 Earls Terrace
London W8 6LP
Helps women with gynaecological problems and dysfunction including PMS and menopause. Write with SAE.

Index